THE WOMAN MISSING IN THE MIRROR

Mary,

THANK you FOR ALLOWING ME TO
BE A PART OF YOUR JOURNEY

Your Foolproof Guide to Getting Back to the
Best Version of You... Body, Mind and Soul

DEAN MITCHELL

The Woman Missing in the Mirror:
Your Foolproof Guide to Getting Back to the Best Version of You…
Body, Mind and Soul

Edited by Cindy Elavsky cindy@cindyelavsky.com.
Photographer, Kelli Taylor purpletreephotograpy.com
Cover and Interior: Streetlight Graphics

To each of the extraordinary women who found the courage to let me walk alongside them on their journey.

If not for you, I would never have had the fortitude to spread my message and offer this book to the world.

To my children Paris, Gavin, Selene and Xander-

May you find the subtle signs life provides each of us, meant to guide you to your purpose in life.

To receive one of Dean's personalized nutrition programs for FREE just follow these two steps!

First, go to www.DeanPMitchell.com and register to join his rapidly growing community of women who have found the woman missing in the mirror.

Next, simply share a selfie of you with your copy of *The Woman Missing In The Mirror* on your Facebook and or Instagram pages or share this video (vimeo.com/181718968) on your Facebook page. Be sure to tag the author and include the hashtag *#ifoundher* !

CONTENTS

PROLOGUE 7

1: FINDING THE BEAUTY IN YOU 11

2: MIND YOUR MOUTH BECAUSE YOUR
WORDS CREATE YOUR EXPECTATIONS 19

3: STRESS AND WORRY 33

4: TURNING YOUR CHILDREN FROM A
BURDEN TO YOUR BENEFIT 75

5: YOUR FIRST LOUSY DAY 87

6: THE MAGIC INGREDIENT NEEDED
FOR LONGTERM RESULTS 99

7: THE DREADED SCALE 109

8: WHY MY CLIENTS COULDN'T CARE
LESS HOW MANY CALORIES THEY'RE BURNING 127

9: EMOTIONAL TRIGGERS AND THE
TRUE DEVASTATION THEY CAUSE 147

10: PROJECTING TO THE FINISH LINE 167

11: FINAL THOUGHTS TO CARRY WITH YOU 179

ABOUT THE AUTHOR 181

CONNECT WITH THE AUTHOR 185

PROLOGUE

For the better part of 15 years, I have been blessed to work with many clients seeking to make any and every physical change you can think of. More specifically, I have worked primarily with females. I won't try to explain how this came to be because I am not entirely certain myself. What I can tell you is that accidental outcome has allowed me to develop a highly effective set of principles specific to females and the challenges they face. Through working intimately with woman of all ages and backgrounds, each providing her own set of unique challenges, has allowed me to see firsthand what works and what simply does not. I've learned through trial and error what methods produce the right changes when it comes to the female body or, even more important, the female mind! As I mentioned, I have worked side by side with each of these special ladies to help her achieve what she had assumed was out of her reach, what was simply an impossibility. Women make this assumption, in my opinion, by allowing society to dictate what their own personal expectations should be. Society states that under the right set of circumstances, she should simply throw in the towel, metaphorically speaking.

In the case of the woman who decides to start her family and have children, or perhaps it's the woman who is busy building her career — climbing that corporate ladder, if you will — or its simply the woman who is in the later stages of life, despite how different each of these cases are, the one thing that doesn't change is the simple fact that society says you need to give up your personal goals in relation to health and fitness if you find yourself in any of these circumstances. This has become the expectation and therefore, the standard, and it's a tragedy because each of you reading this is capable of so much more. This is why I've developed my unique set of principles and is ultimately how this book came to exist. After meeting hundreds of woman who were hopeless, whose self-esteem and self-worth where nowhere to be found, whose expectations for themselves and how they should look and feel had reached an all-time low, it had become just what society says it should. I decided to focus my energy and efforts to developing a solution to this epidemic.

Despite the gratification I receive from watching dramatic physical transformations in each and every one of the amazing women I work with, there is a far more rewarding gift each of them has unintentionally given me. They take me on a journey of personal experiences they never dreamed possible. I get to watch a wife rekindle the flame with her spouse after twenty years of marriage by looking into the mirror and finding that confident, healthy, sexy woman that just a short time ago was only a distant memory occasionally glanced at through old wedding photos hanging on the wall. Or I get to experience the joy a grandmother gets when she's able to hike up a mountain with her grandkids for the first time. That same mountain that the year prior forced her to disappoint her grandkids as she told them she couldn't make the trip up, saying, "It's just too far and I am too old!" I get to witness all the priceless lessons a mother teaches her child or children as she shows them firsthand how to stay strong and persevere, how to set and reach new goals, and how to let nothing stand in the way of her potential. Most important, I get to watch each and every one of these special ladies who first sat down in my office broken and defeated, filled with self-doubt, depression and hopelessness, grow into the highly confident, highly capable woman she is today, the woman I could see below the surface the second she walked into my office!

My hope is that you'll apply the same principles found in this book to create whoever you wish to see staring back at you when you look in the mirror. That you get to experience the highest level of your physical potential regardless of your circumstances, just as each of my clients has. I have included all of the foundational principles I use with each and every one of my female clients, regardless of age or fitness level. These are tools that can be applied at no cost and used for the rest of your life. They can be applied in any setting and under any circumstance. Trust me when I say I have yet to find a woman whom the principles in this book did not help drastically.

"A rose can never be a sunflower, and a sunflower can never be a rose. All flowers are beautiful in their own way and that's like women too."

—Miranda Kerr

1:

FINDING THE BEAUTY IN YOU

When I initially sit down with a woman to discuss her fitness goals, I have a set of key questions I often lead with. These are questions that help to give me a better perspective of where I need to start when designing her program — or, at least, that's what she is thinking! Although it is true that those questions are useful and in most cases needed in regard to qualifying her physical state, there is a much bigger process taking place. I am working to get a glimpse into her state of mind. I find with almost certainty that there is a profound connection between a woman's desire to see physical improvements in the mirror and a deeper underlying struggle in her mental perspective, in how she perceives herself.

Though it took me years in my career before I was able to make the connection, I finally started noting that how a woman views herself — who she sees in the mirror — can be and often times is drastically different than how she is actually perceived by others. Now for those of you thinking, "No news flash there," I bring up this point to reflect on the fact that this is a true statement in some regard with every single female client I have worked with to date. In speaking with a potential client, I would pick up subtle little comments or self-directed jokes during our initial conversations that were made to be comical but could quickly be seen as her true perspective of herself, regardless of age, social status or current physical state.

The fact that no matter who I was talking to, no matter how confident or successful she was, despite the uniqueness of each woman, they all shared this same disposition. The realization of this was truly profound in my work and ultimately my abilities to help whoever she was, which I will discuss in later chapters.

Making this connection was quite bizarre to me. To think that the majority of women walking around in the world shared this view or feeling of inadequacy. This was challenging for me to understand, but after spending some time thinking about it, it began to make complete sense. I will help to illustrate how with an analogy.

You hold in your possession two paintings. One happens to be the world's most expensive painting, priceless and irreplaceable; the other is a cheap knockoff of that same painting that holds no monetary value by comparison. By human nature, your actions with the priceless version would be to handle it with extreme care, making sure to protect it and keep it safe at all times, as you should. After all, it's only logical if you possess something considered priceless and irreplaceable! Now in the case of the other painting, the cheap knockoff, despite the fact that it shares a distinct resemblance, the fact still remains you will more than likely handle it with little regard or care, with ultimately no concern for what happens to it because, after all, it's worthless and can be replaced at relatively no cost, right?

I told you this story to help illustrate what virtually every woman has struggled with when they initially sit down with me. The perspective that they are in fact the cheap knockoff version of that priceless painting! Keeping this perspective in the back of your mind, it becomes easy to see how a woman would struggle to make any real commitments to her own self-improvement. That's not to say that when she looks in the mirror and is not pleased with what she sees, she doesn't wish for physical changes, but again, being the cheap knockoff that holds no true value, why would she make any investment in herself? It is this mindset that is the driving force behind what keeps a woman from dedicating herself to her capabilities and ultimately her results.

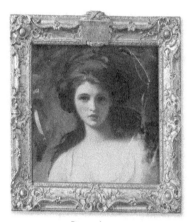
Priceless

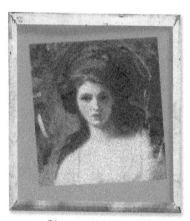
Cheap Knock Off

Addressing this mindset is the initial task I place upon myself, and I work to immediately overcome, in most cases, depending on the individual and just how skewed her view is. As I already mentioned, in my earlier career I struggled to see just how important this part of the process was. I would often find that I was applying the same practices and attention to all of my clients, having some reach the highest levels of their physical potential with little struggle, if any, while others would progress with minimal results, at best, and ultimately throw in the towel on reaching their goals. Although some trainers would simply move on to the next client, I found myself compelled to understand what the missing link was, why the practices that achieve such success with most would be a complete flop with others. This puzzled and frustrated me for years to come until I was blessed with a few key clients. Keeping them nameless for privacy, my opportunity to work with them would forever change how I worked with female clients and members moving forward.

The few key women I am referring to started with just one, who, after seeing tremendous success quickly, became a walking billboard for me and my unique program. This was followed up quickly with her friends jumping on the bandwagon shortly after.

Now I need to bring a couple of key pieces of information into the story at this point to best illustrate things. Being a business owner in a very affluent community, it is not uncommon to have women who would be considered physically attractive, oftentimes holding high-level positions in large companies, coming in and out of my facility. These are women who society would place into the category of highly functioning and highly successful individuals. I don't make this point to pay them a compliment through a book, but rather to give the reader the proper visual perspective of them. My view of them during initial introductions was that they would be confident and comfortable in their skin. On occasion I would even catch myself intimidated by the woman sitting across from me with her beauty or personal achievements. Through initial conversations, however, I was shocked to quickly learn that no matter the level of her beauty, success or social status, the majority of these woman when looking in the mirror saw the cheap knockoff painting. How could this be possible? I suppose it was that very question that led me to the discoveries that ultimately changed the way I handled all my female clients from that point on.

I feel that my approach to reaching fitness goals with my clients is unique from most others because I teach them the importance of valuing themselves. This is not to say you need to become egotistical or self-centered, but understanding your true beauty is, in my opinion, a must. This one single concept has laid the foundation of my work and transcends through all aspects of the service I provide to my clients on a daily basis.

TESTIMONIAL

I am a 46 year old mother of four. I had decided at the age 40 that I wanted to get healthy! I worked out non stop for 5 years and tried just about every program you could imagine. This along with a healthy diet, at least at the time what I thought was healthy. At one point I even gave up all alcohol for 8 months thinking maybe that was the culprit. Over the years I was noticing positive changes but just not significant enough for all my hard work. I decided it was time to try one more program. That is when I met Dean Mitchell and everything changed! I remember telling him that he was my last hope to get the results I had been dreaming of and that if I didn't after giving my all I was giving up.

It was at our first consultation that he sat me down and started asking me questions about my goals, daily nutrition intake and timing along with exercise schedule. With that information alone he immediately told me he could help and WOW did he! The way he explained it to me was basically that I had been starving my self and working out too much.. which went against everything that my generation, especially woman were taught. Dean set me up on different variations of nutrition schedules which ran a course of a couple weeks for each. I was eating more food than I ever thought possible, and was eating anywhere from 5 to 7 meals a day. Throughout the different stages he was always there for support and help with any questions I had. He measured me monthly to check my progress and would adjust whenever needed to help me reach the goal that I had set. Not only did I reach my goal but then set new ones. I competed in my first figure competition with his support, something I have never thought in a million years I would ever be capable of. Not only does he give you the knowledge to reach your goals, but healthy habits for a lifetime!! It doesn't matter your age, your lifestyle or your schedule, if your willing to put in the effort and dedication, Dean will get you the results your after with his knowledge!! I have now been a member of his gym and program for almost two years and can't imagine ever leaving.

Sincerely Yvonne

We know what we are, but know not what we may be.

—William Shakespeare

2:

MIND YOUR MOUTH BECAUSE YOUR WORDS CREATE YOUR EXPECTATIONS

No, I am not referring to your choice in words when you accidentally stub your toe on the corner of the hallway while chasing your naked two-year-old to finish his or her diaper install. I am referring to a much bigger mistake that was being made by virtually all of my clients before starting with me that unfortunately comes at a high price. Allow me to explain by starting off with an exercise I want you to participate in right now. I want you to create a small list of just five habitual words or phrases that you use to illustrate the way you feel when placed in the following two scenarios.

Create your first list based on simply standing in front of the mirror. What are the first descriptive words that come to mind? What are the five habitual words or phrases you use when you see your reflection in the mirror? Some of you might even feel such strong emotional attachment to them that you actually speak them out loud unintentionally. Write them down, and be sure to take your time and answer truthfully. Also, be sure to remember we are looking for habitual words and phrases or, in other words, ones that are used most frequently, not just on occasion. Using the same set of rules, let's start a brand-new list and apply it to this next scenario.

You have plans for a night out on the town with a small group of your closest girlfriends at a favorite local hangout. In preparation for your night out, you decide to keep things low-key and opt for something semi-casual from the closet, nothing out of the ordinary or too over the top. You neither do anything special with your hair nor do you change the way you applied your makeup. Upon arriving, you spot your friends and are greeted with the textbook "hello" behavior that so many of you are famous for. It's sure to include lots of hugs, kisses to cheeks, and heightened levels of excitement while saying the words, "Hi!" or "Hello!" However, this time, something else is included, something you weren't expecting. Each of your friends can't get over how great you look since they last saw you and make it a point to tell you this, showering you with compliments. They keep referring to how much smaller you have gotten or how great your pants look on you. This comes as a shock to you even though you've been much more diligent with your diet and exercise lately. In this scenario, how do you respond? More important, what are some of the key habitual words or phases you use as internal dialogue in those responses? I stress the term "internal" because I have learned it's not uncommon for a woman to say one thing while they think another in these situations. Oftentimes saying things out loud like, "Oh, you're too kind. Stop it" or "You really think so?" or even just reply with a simple "Thank you." All this while inside they are thinking, "Oh my god, have I actually gotten fatter and they think a compliment will make me feel better?" or "OK, why are they sucking up to me, something must be wrong?" or just a simple "My outfit must look terrible and they just don't want to be rude by saying so!"

I won't claim to know what you're thinking or put words in your mouth, but I can say with a high level of certainty from watching interactions between members at my gym or my own interactions with personal clients, your list probably includes the following choices in habitual words or phrases. In the case of your list you created when looking in the mirror, you probably included words or phrases like:

- DISGUSTING
- FAT
- OUT OF SHAPE
- I WILL NEVER CHANGE
- I DON'T LOOK ANY DIFFERENT

In the case of the list created from your night out on the town with your girls and all of them telling you how much you have changed physically and how great your clothes look on you, your list might include the following:

- THEY ARE CRAZY
- THEY MUST BE LYING TO ME
- I MUST LOOK REALLY BAD AND THEY ARE TRYING TO MAKE ME FEEL BETTER
- SOMEONE MUST HAVE SOME BAD NEWS TO SHARE WITH ME

I had you do this exercise to make this section of my book as personal as possible. I did this with the hope of driving home the importance of applying the tools we are about to discuss and reversing the habit of using the wrong words or phrases on a daily basis.

How many of you reading this have heard the saying "Thoughts become things"? Well in the event you haven't, I guarantee you have applied this concept a time or two in your life, perhaps daily in the event that you're a parent like I am. I will define the phrase "Thoughts become things" as "Whatever your expectation is for any given situation often dictates what your outcome will be."

Take the example of my twelve-year-old daughter during her first swim meet. She was petrified, literally lying in the fetal position on a grassy hillside off to the side of pool area. She lay there for every bit of thirty minutes, refusing to swim, let alone move, due to stomach pain. She described the pain as something tearing her stomach in two from the inside out. Like something you would expect out of the movie *Alien*. All of this despite the fact that for the weeks leading up her big meet, she couldn't have been more anxious or excited to compete. I had a hunch it was just anxiety from the arrival of her big day, but just to be safe, I put my EMT license to good use and performed a quick abdominal assessment, thankfully finding no alien or issues to be present.

With a strong personal belief in the idea that our thoughts truly do dictate our abilities and outcomes, I knew I had to do something other than simply force her to swim. I knew I had to get her to shift gears mentally; I had to get her to shift back to that state of excitement, back to that state of being filled with so much positive energy from the thought of swimming in her first meet that she could hardly contain herself waiting for the day to finally arrive.

The fact that she is a brilliant little girl, fully capable of functioning at an extremely high cognitive level, meant she is also fully capable of rationalizing with the fact that she made a commitment to her team, not to mention all of us who chose to support her and drive an hour to watch her on her big day. However, by simply demanding she swim under principles of logic, I would have effectively set her up for failure long before her hands ever touched the water. Even knowing what she should do in terms of right and wrong, without the proper state of mind behind her actions, she would have, at best, put in minimal effort, equipped with the expectation she was going to perform terribly, that she would surely be doomed to fail.

Luckily for us, all the stars aligned that day, and with help from me, her mother and her swim coaches, she made the decision independently to swim in the meet that day and see just what she was capable of. Needless to say, I was proud to watch her take that leap of faith off the block into the water and give it her all, and it turned out to be a memory that will never leave me — she ended up beating the rest of the competition and winning her race!

This story is an example of a mistake I see new members make time and time again. They show up for their workout with the wrong mindset. They show up with no actual interest in the level of intensity they are going to apply. Instead they are just hoping the hour passes by as quickly as possible so they can carry on with the list of more enjoyable activities they have planned for that day. I know this to be true because I hear them discussing what the rest of their day entails while they are lunging up and down the workout floor. Discussing the latest sale at the local boutique while they are pressing dumbbells over their heads. Now I am not saying you should not make friends at your local gym or engage in conversations. I am proud to say we have developed a culture in my facility that has breed friendships that will last a lifetime. I am simply stating you might be more benefited to save the conversations for the right time, perhaps during a recovery period or water break.

I cannot stress enough the effects that just simply concentrating during your workout will have on the result you see in the mirror, a skill I work tirelessly to cultivate with every single member who walks through our doors. The quality of the work you're able to put in during exercise will provide qualities you never dreamed possible in the mirror. I believe this to be so true that I have been known to stop a group training session in its tracks if I find that group of ladies seems to be particularly chatty that day. I do this with a quick shout-out asking them to stop right where they are. I go around the room, asking each of them individually if they are focusing on that squat I asked them to perform and the key fundamentals needed while performing it. I ask the first girl if she is focusing on making sure the pressure is in her heels, as it should be. Then I ask the next if she is keeping her toes pointed up to the ceiling in her shoes to ensure she keeps that pressure back in heels consistently. Then the next girl if she is squeezing her glutes at the top of her motion, or if she's simply moving up and down, waiting for me to call time on that set. Then the next if she is focusing on her tempo, making sure not to move too fast on the way down or too slow on the way up. It's easy to see how lack of focus could very well limit your ability to perform exercises correctly and ultimately leave you less then pleased when looking in the mirror. To think, some wonder why their success is moderate at best. Now let's look at it from the perspective or mindset I work so intensely to develop in each of the ladies who work with me. The moment any of them walk in that front door, they know it is time to set everything else aside and focus on their results. Each of those ladies knows it's time to focus on achieving the results her body is already designed and ready to create. She knows that hour spent working out is a simple conversation between herself and her body asking for the changes she wants to see. It is in knowing this that the focus and hard work required for her body to respond is created and applied.

Perhaps apply the idea of thoughts becoming things to your own child or children. We have all had the occasional talk with our little ones at some point reminding them of how special they are, how they in fact do not have an extremely low IQ in the event they received a poor test grade in school. We work to constantly reinforce how they are capable of anything and everything they want out of life. Why do we do that as parents? We do it because we consciously or subconsciously know that if our child walks around thinking they are not special in every way, not as capable in every way or less intelligent, they run the risk of believing it. They run the risk of that skewed view becoming their reality, ultimately letting it dictate the decisions they make and the effort they put in, as so many of us do as adults.

Referring back to your two lists you created, do any of your habitual words or phrases consistently used by you in either scenario provide you with positive reinforcement, or is it perhaps the opposite situation? Are you, on a consistent basis, breaking yourself down? Are you, on a consistent basis, reminding yourself of how awful you look or feel? Can you see how this habit destroys any opportunity of your actually achieving the level of success you're so desperate for when looking in the mirror, the level of success that requires the focus and dedication I just described to you? After all, who is going to maintain the motivation needed to stay focused or dedicated to anything if all they hear day in and day out is how they are failing, they aren't making any progress, they are fat, or they are out of shape? No one, myself included, would stick to or stay dedicated to a goal with that kind of negative reinforcement attached to it.

Those of you who are saying, "OK, this is all fine and great, but I am also not delusional. The habitual words or phrases from my list are how I really feel deep down inside and therefore can't be changed." I strongly disagree! I personally believed in the validity of my thoughts and their impact on me long before I started applying it to fitness or how I work with clients. I have stumbled upon proof of the effects of thoughts becoming things in not only my personal life, but also through a long list of books and authors such as Paulo Coelho and his book titled The *Alchemist* or Dr. Wayne Dyer and his book titled *How to Be a No-Limit Person*, as well as Tony Robbins and his book titled *Awakening the Giant Within*, just to reference a few.

It wasn't until during reading one of Robbins' books that I was able to make a significant connection to a principle that I had been applying for years in both my personal and business life. Despite the fact I had discovered this method years prior and understood it's importance, I had not yet put my finger on exactly what I was doing, not until stumbling upon Robbins' application of it. You see, I knew beyond a doubt there was a drastic difference between what my internal dialogue would sound like in either of the scenarios I gave earlier when I asked you to create your list of habitual words and phrases. In Robbins' book, he describes a term called "Transformational Vocabulary," which is basically defined that through changing your habitual vocabulary, you hold the ability to transform your experience.

Let's both pull out our lists of habitual words and phrases, and see firsthand how transformational vocabulary applies. In the scenario of looking in the mirror, while your key word or phrase might be "out of shape" or "fat," I might be saying to myself, "I am not there yet, but I will make more progress today" or "I am going to reduce my midsection a little more today." In the scenario of friends paying a compliment to me about how much tighter my midsection looks, even in the event I don't see the changes they are referring to when I look in the mirror, I don't assume they are crazy or lying to me. Instead I have taught myself to feel excited by the fact that someone else is noticing my hard work, especially in the case where I never brought it up. I know this is proof that my hard work is paying off. As discussed in other sections of this book, I understand that because I see myself on a daily basis, it is completely normal to overlook physical changes because they happen at such a gradual rate. Understanding this fact allows me to accept a metaphorical pat on the back from another human being when they are trying to give it, an action so many of us fail to include in our daily routines out of fear of being considered egotistical or conceited. The irony is that one compliment we so quickly force ourselves to disregard and set aside has within it more power than any fat burner, diet or piece of equipment you'll find in a gym. It has the power to keep you motivated and on track, just as your compliments do for your children.

When looking at it from this perspective, you can see how

your list can be seen as destructive or counterproductive in nature. While mine doesn't reflect that I am necessarily satisfied, it doesn't make the results I am looking for seem that out of reach. A statement like, "I am going to reduce my midsection a little more today" can be interpreted as I still have some changes that need to take place, but I am fully capable and am taking steps closer to my end goal every day. It is easy to see how my inner dialogue is both deliberate and empowering.

Those of you who are at this point finding this to be a somewhat delusional approach, I will offer one more example of a child who is struggling with schoolwork or perhaps self-esteem. I would bet if this were your child, the last thing you would tell them to do is stand in front of a mirror while you tell them they are ugly, they are fat or that they are unintelligent, but yet so many of you do this exact thing to yourself. So many of you stand in front of that mirror berating the woman who's looking back: You tell her how disgusting she is, how fat or out of shape she is and, even worse, you tell her how she's not even worth the time and energy to change it! Why on Earth would you do that to yourself?

I wrote this book in an effort to ask you to make the commitment to stop this behavior immediately! I promise you, you're worth it! Make a game out of it. Take those lists you wrote out with your habitual words or phrases, and next to each one, right down a word or phrase that would be considered empowering and positive. You don't even have to actually believe it at this stage, just humor me and write it down. You can steal the examples I provided earlier if you wish to, but make sure that once you have created the positive empowering side of your list, you commit to using it immediately. It will take some practice, without question, but every time you catch yourself starting that same old internal dialogue you have used for as long as you can remember, stop immediately and start to play the game. Replace your usual "Oh my gosh, I am still so fat" with "I think I will lose some more inches today." Delusional or not, this gets your brain to let go of the visual image that you're fat and always will be and replaces it with a vision that you're not yet at your goal, but you're losing inches while you're looking in the mirror! The application of this principle shifts you into a mental position of doing rather than complaining, and reinforcing the fact that you're not happy in some way, shape or form. This gets your mind to paint the visual picture of exactly what you're looking for in the mirror. This is the mental state that I and all of my clients operate in at all times.

This is the mental state that allows us to focus our energy and efforts on the solution rather than the problem, a key fundamental that so many women are missing.

So be delusional, make it fun and make it a game — be your own biggest fan! Go back to being that little girl who isn't afraid to take a compliment when it's given. Don't be robbed of all the joys you're meant to experience along the way by telling yourself you're not allowed to do so until you've reached your goal. It is your ability to collect and hold onto all the little moments of gratitude that will allow you to reach physical transformations you never dreamed possible.

TESTIMONIAL

My name is Devin and I am twenty-three years old. My journey with Dean Mitchell began about three months ago after I had graduated college. I have always been an active person, however my diet and nutrition would get in the way of the results I truly hoped to achieve. To put it frankly, I started his program due to the fact that I didn't have much to lose, but SO much to gain.

My goal was not to lose weight per say, but to gain muscle as well as knowledge pertaining to diet and nutrition. I wanted to learn what to put into my body and at what times in order to see the results I have been craving for the past several years. The program is changing my life in several ways. As stated before I am learning how to eat properly in order to maintain and grow muscle, while at the same time deteriorating unwanted fat. The group training I attend at his gym assists me and force me to challenge my body into forming muscles and building strength in places I never knew I could. The support I am given on a daily basis, not only from Dean but the other individuals that attend his facility is truly motivating and inspiring. I have already seen and felt such an improvement with my body and emotional state. Every time I attend a session at Mitchell Fitness Solutions I amaze myself at how much stronger I get every time. Dean Mitchell has honestly changed my life, and continues to every single day.

Sincerely Devin

Worrying does not empty tomorrow of its troubles. It empties today of its strength.

—*Mary Engelrein*

3:
STRESS AND WORRY

OK, ladies, this is not an attempt to throw you into some kind of a self-help book or make the claim that I am some kind of positivity guru. However, this will prove to be an important chapter because it contains some of my most fundamental principles used by every single one of my clients.

I won't claim to know what it feels like to walk in your shoes and deal with some of the challenges each of you do. I won't make the statement that a challenging situation you're being faced with should have no effect on you or be disregarded. I am simply asking you to take a deep breath, take a step back, and ask yourself if whatever it is that's getting the best of you is improved or solved by you worrying or stressing about it? Do worry and stress make your challenging situation or metaphorical rock in the road seem smaller or larger? If you're answering any of these questions after removing the emotions you've attached to the hurdle you're faced with, the answer is most definitely, "No, my choice to worry or stress is not making that rock in the road any smaller, its only making it bigger by the second!"

I bring this point up to touch on the key principle of removing the emotions you attach to any challenging situation you feel might hinder your ability to stay on your fitness journey. We'll touch on this in other chapters and how it's oftentimes easier said than done to think only with the rational side of your brain all the time. To clarify, I am not asking you to do that all the time because I think that is not humanly possible. We all have days that are worse than others or are put into situations that leave us feeling down and out. I am simply saying that how you initially respond doesn't have to be your final response. Let me give you an example. Let's say you find yourself in a small fender bender. You were rear-ended by a young teenager who clearly needed a few more hours in driver's training. No one was injured and the damage was minimal. Despite the fact that it was an accident — after all, who would intentionally rear-end another car? — you're still angry that you now have to deal with this fiasco and go through all the insurance hoops we all know too well.

Despite the fact that your initial reaction was to become angered by the situation you had no control over, it's the choice you make next that will dictate if the rest of your experience with this situation will go smoothly or become a huge burden. You have to choose if you're going to continue to react to this situation with anger or if you're going to think rationally and remind yourself that accidents happen and being angry will not change the situation. For those of you who are saying to yourself, "This guy's delusional. If it were that easy, everyone would do it. He must have lived an extremely sheltered life. If he only knew what it feels like to try to function like a normal human being, let alone try to stay on a diet or follow a workout regimen when you're dealing with real-life problems!" let me share a little bit of my background with you.

I have been told through conversations with my closest friends and clients that my real background and what they expect it to be are two very different things. Most think I came from wealth and good fortune. That I came from a home filled with lots of love and two caring parents who reflected the definition of a perfect marriage. This, however, is not how my story was written. I have experienced more real-life problems as described earlier in the thirty-four years I've been on this Earth than most will experience in a lifetime.

It started with being the outcome of a one-night stand my mother had in the younger years of her life. At a time in her life when she struggled to take care of herself, let alone a new baby, she suffered from both manic depression and bipolar disorder. She was twenty years old when she gave birth to me and was still struggling with drug and alcohol addiction. Although it's been said she was clean during her pregnancy with me, and I would like to think so, I cannot be certain. As anyone who has dealt with a family member or friend who struggles with addiction knows, being truthful is not a prescribed practice. Unfortunately this was also a time in my mother's life when she was somewhat promiscuous, resulting in some confusion as to who my father actually was. The end result was my birth certificate reflecting the last name of a man who turned out to be the wrong person based on the features (blond hair, green eyes and short height) that I grew into.

By the time this was discovered, my real father had relocated and wasn't found until many years later (around my eighteenth birthday, to be exact) through mine and my mother's efforts. This task unfortunately proved to be uneventful because he had no interest in a relationship with me. I had no knowledge until the age of eight that the man who I thought was my father wasn't my birth father until my mother decided to tell me the truth that her husband at the time was not my real father and that my younger sister and brother were only my half-siblings. Despite the initial shock and confusion I am sure any eight year old would experience in that situation, I found myself relieved by the thought that I shared no real connection to her husband. I didn't particularly care for him. He was a man who stood around six feet tall with a stocky build and tattoos he had acquired from his many stints in and out of prison. He had been arrested for everything from robbery to rape. He too suffered from drug and alcohol addiction and suffered from bipolar disorder as well. I honestly have very few memories of him due to a natural coping mechanism I am sure I developed at a young age. I will tell you it was not the most loving environment for me or my siblings.

Now, being a grown adult, it is easy for me to pinpoint what were contributing factors to the constant fighting and tension in the little apartment we lived in at the time. I can recall one time in particular that my mother had kicked him out of the house, for what reason I can't recall. The next day he waited for us to leave and broke into the house and stole all of our food from both the refrigerator and pantry. I can still picture the look of panic on my mother's face as we pulled up to find the glass panel adjacent to our front door shattered, with broken glass everywhere. I remember keeping my two younger siblings, who must have been around the ages of two and five, locked in the car with me, fearful that whoever had done this was still in our house. After my mother had discovered what actually happened, she was both frantic and hysterical because at the time, we were on welfare, and she had no other resources to feed the four of us.

Up to this point in my life, I had always spent time during the week living with my grandparents. I don't recall how this circumstance came to be, but I think it was greatly due to the fact that when I was born, my mother was still living with them and dependent on their support. I think it was only natural for them to take over in the areas of parenting where she struggled. This, coupled with the fact that my mother's decisions to still continue the use of drugs and alcohol rather than be a parent to her brand-new baby, gave them no choice but to step in when and where they could. This allowed a bond to develop between us that would rival any child's bond with his or her biological parents, and proved to be one of the most valuable gifts I would ever receive.

To this day I couldn't tell you why, but unfortunately, this same bond was never developed between my younger siblings and grandparents. This oftentimes forced me to leave them behind during the time I spent with my grandparents. This was really hard for me because I knew my life was so different with my grandparents, and I wanted to share it with my sister and brother but never could. Don't let me confuse you: My grandparents were blue-collar and lived a very modest life by most people's standards. We lived in a smaller home — I would guess around twelve-hundred square feet in Huntington Beach, California, the southern part of the state. My grandfather (who I now refer to as Dad) worked as a mechanic, while my grandmother worked as a hairstylist. Both jobs paid modest salaries and left us with a tight budget at times, but I had my own room with a closet filled with clothes, I had toys and a bike to ride through a safe neighborhood — things I was not so accustomed to when at mom's house.

By comparison my life with my mother and two siblings was entirely different. Prior to my stepfather coming into the picture when I was eleven, my sister, Ashlee, was seven and our little brother, Tyler, was five, our life was different than most other kids our age. I can recall the three of us sharing a room and a single mattress at one point in time. As I mentioned, we depended on the welfare system for our food, so staples in our house — which I am not ashamed to say, I still love to this day — always included ramen noodles and a dish my mom used to make called chip beef on toast. Both of these were extremely economical meals for her to make and feed three hungry little mouths with. We obviously didn't have much extra money, so going out to restaurants or doing leisure activities together, like going to see a movie, didn't happen very often.

I will always remember one of the special treats my mom would often allow for, one that the three of us always looked forward to. At the time, the area of Southern California that we lived in was home to a large Spanish community. One of the members of that community was a gentleman who made his living walking up and down the streets of Costa Mesa, the city we lived in, offering a simple snack that would prove to be a part of my childhood I would never forget. His clothes were tattered, leaving no question as to the fact he had more then likely purchased them from the local Salvation Army. His shoes were dirty and worn from the miles he put on them daily. He was an older man, with hands that reflected his age and all the years of hard work he must have used them for. To anyone who didn't know any better, he could have easily been mistaken for a homeless man. It was clear he didn't have much money and had more then likely struggled through hardship the majority of his life. Despite this, I remember him always smiling. Regardless if it was the beginning of his day and he was just getting started or the end of it when he has surely walked twenty miles at least, pushing a heavy shopping cart and serving up his unique snack.

He walked the streets with a makeshift food cart that he fashioned from an old, abandoned grocery cart with wheels you could hear squeaking long before he appeared. His cart was filled with only a few items. A large metal pot that he kept full with fresh corn and the hot water it was boiled in, oftentimes seeping steam from its lid as he made his way slowly down the sidewalk. Next to the pot sat a cardboard box filled with the other ingredients needed to create our favorite treats growing up. He would pull from his metal pot a wonderful piece of bright yellow corn, while reaching in his cardboard box of goodies for the butter and mayonnaise with which he used to slather up the corn. He would then coat it with a generous sprinkling of Parmesan cheese and paprika, and wrap in wax paper as if it were a burrito. As simple as this sounds, it is absolutely delicious, and just the thought of it brings me back to special moments in time. With the level of poverty we lived in, this was our trip to the candy store. This was our family trip to a fine restaurant, and we were overjoyed because of it.

Despite the constant concern I carried around with me for my sister and brother's wellbeing while I was away, my relationship with my grandparents continued to grow and flourish. This resulted in my decision to have my last name legally changed to theirs. With no idea who my real father was, it made more sense to share the last name of the man who I now consider my father.

Eventually my mom divorced from my siblings' father, found love again, and eventually became married to one of the greatest men I have come to know. A man who, to this day, is committed to her despite a marriage plagued with drug and alcohol relapses and struggles with mental disorders. At the age of fifteen, I moved out of my mother's house and permanently into my grandparents', where life was good. I had gone from continually fighting with my mother over her constant struggles to stay clean and make better decisions to the consistent support and positive reinforcement my grandmother had always provided. She always made it a point to remind me of how special I was, how I was capable of anything, and I was going to do something great with myself. Although at the time I laughed it off and didn't take her statements too seriously, I can now see how she was planting a seed that would allow me to grow into the person I am today.

Unfortunately at the age of eighteen things would change drastically for me. The woman who had stepped in to play such a pivotal role in my life, the woman who had taught me it was OK to believe her when she said she loved me more than any drug and would always be there for me, the woman who I had come to think of as my anchor that I could use to weather even the worst storms was diagnosed with stage-four small-cell lung cancer and given only six months to live. After a visit to the doctor's office for what she assumed was just a nasty cough she couldn't seem to shake, the test results showed it was much worse.

I remember standing in the hospital room by her bedside when the doctor came in with the diagnoses. I remember the feeling of struggling to breathe, as if someone had wrapped their hands around my throat and was slowly squeezing tighter and tighter as the doctor told me I would have only six more months with her. This was the first real feeling of loss I had experienced. I had suffered tragedies and tough times, like the time I shattered my right femur into eight pieces from a dirt-bike crash and was told I might not walk again. Even that experience would not prepare me for the news I received that day. The months following were spent helping my grandmother adjust to her new life filled with doctors appointments, medication and painful procedures, often leaving her ill and to weak to walk. Despite the fact that we all wanted to be optimistic, I could see in her eyes that she knew her life on Earth with me would soon come to an end, and I wanted to help take away the pain of that reality in any way possible.

With my grandfather being the main source of income, he had to keep working, requiring me to tend to her needs. My usual activities in the months leading up to her passing were grocery shopping, preparing meals for her and my grandfather, and keeping up on the household chores. Driving her to and from doctors' appointments was also something I was tasked with. My grandfather did what he could, but at this stage an average workweek for him often added up to between eighty and ninety hours. I remember doing surprisingly well with the whole situation, at least in the beginning. It wasn't until the final months of her life, when the disease had begun to affect her brain, that I found myself really struggling. This was a hard experience for me to try to process even at nineteen, an age when most are considered adults. I will never forget that look of confusion reflecting back through her green eyes because she no longer knew who the person was smiling back at her. She no longer knew me as her son, as that little boy she so many years before sheltered from circumstances no child should go through. I was nothing more than a stranger now.

It was around this point that my grandfather opted for hospice to assist us with her on a daily basis. This allowed us to keep her with us for her final journey home. I still remember it as if it had happened yesterday. Hospice came as they did daily to check all her vitals and tend to any of her other needs. On this particular day, though, her vitals showed it was her time to go. They let me, my grandfather and my uncle know that it was time to say our goodbyes. I remember feeling reluctant to say anything to her because I knew it would be the most difficult thing I had ever done, and the rational side of me figured she wouldn't hear my words at this stage anyway. My emotional side told me that if I didn't say that final goodbye and tell her I loved her one more time before she was gone, it would be something I would regret for the rest of my life. It was from that thought that I found the strength I needed. As she lay there with her eyes closed and her breathing becoming more and more labored from her body shutting down, I leaned down to her ear and whispered my last words to her: "I am so thankful you were a part of my life; you didn't have to be. I love you. It's OK to go home now." After doing so, the three of us stood by her bedside, my uncle and I each holding one of her hands while my grandfather rubbed her head, offering what comfort we could as she took her last breath. I remember after she had passed and hospice came back to collect her thinking this has to be the worst thing I will experience in my life, losing the woman who was essentially my mother before I was even out of my teens. Sadly, I was wrong, and it proved to only be the prelude for what was to come.

> *The tragedy of life is not death… but what we let die inside of us while we live.*
>
> *—Norman Cousins*

My next brush with troublesome times came in the form of a massive stroke that would leave my mother completely paralyzed on one side of her body at the young age of forty-four. Her initial diagnosis was that the injuries sustained to her brain from the stroke would prove to be fatal or at best leave her in a vegetative state. Aside from the obvious reasons that this would be a traumatic experience for everyone involved, it could not have happened at a worse time because it had been several weeks since my mother and I had spoken due to an argument between the two of us, an argument that left me disowned and reminded of how she thought of me as one of the bigger mistakes she had ever made — something that was more common in our relationship then I would like to admit. I am told this is part of what is to be expected from someone suffering from manic depression and bipolar disorder, but I can't say it made the experience anymore tolerable. Despite the fact that the last time my mother spoke to me she made it clear she wanted it to be the last, despite the anger and frustration I still felt toward her, deep down I still loved her unconditionally and rushed to her bedside as soon as I got the news of what had happened.

Upon arriving at the emergency room of our local hospital, I was greeted by my stepfather, who had been pacing up and down the hallway. He quickly brought me up to speed. He informed me that her stroke was caused by a blood vessel that burst, causing a massive bleed. The head of the hospital's neurological department had informed him that he unfortunately would not be able to repair the vessel because it was located in an area of her brain that would cause more damage than benefit by going into. This was the point he told us she had a fifty percent chance of surviving, and if she did, it was highly probable she would spend the rest of her life in full paralysis, not even capable of breathing on her own.

The months to follow were spent in the hospital by her side. She was placed in the intensive-care unit in a medically induced coma to allow her brain to better heal with minimal activity. I remember sitting in the room with her listening to the machines breathing for her. She was filled with what I assumed was every tube and device the hospital carried. There were tubes coming out of her arms and legs to help with circulation. There were more tubes coming out of her nose, mouth and throat to help her breath. Lastly, there were more tubes coming out of her head to relieve the pressure on her brain by draining excess fluid. I remember sitting in a chair down by her feet that was angled to face her and looking up at her lifeless body. I remember thinking that despite all the pain she had caused in my life, all the times she had hurt me with her words, all the times she let me down, all the times she made me feel unwanted and worthless, I still wished I could take her pain away. I still wished I could talk to her one more time to tell her that no matter what, I would always love her.

I recall pulling out my phone to listen to a message she had left on my voicemail only days before. I sat there in that dark room with her and nothing but the sound of a ventilator breathing for her, listening to that voicemail just so I could hear her voice again. A voicemail that days before I couldn't bring myself to play all the way through because it was too painful to listen to. She had left it after our fight, and it was intended to inform me that I was no longer her son and to not contact her again. Looking back on it, I would have probably been wiser to not listen to a voicemail like that under that set of circumstances, but I knew it was highly likely that I would never hear her voice again, that I would never get the chance to speak to her again. I was willing to take anything I could get. Luckily I was wrong, and my mother pulled through after the better part of two full months in intensive care. Although we are extremely grateful for it, as I mentioned earlier, she had been left with paralysis down one entire side of her body and a severe inability to articulate her words, making it very challenging at times to communicate with her. As time goes by, her mental functions continue to decline as well. Although I will never have the ability to share normal life experiences with my mother, I am grateful to still have her around to this day.

By the time of my mother's stroke, I was more independent than my younger siblings, who were both still living at home with my parents. I was twenty-four, which would have put my sister at twenty and brother at eighteen. Knowing my siblings were both more dependent on my mother than I was left me concerned for how they would cope with her no longer being there for them. This concern would prove to be a valid one in the years to come.

At this stage in my life, I found myself lost and confused as to why I was put in the position I was. I had no idea how to pick up the pieces left behind from the tragedies of losing a woman I thought of as my mother at nineteen to learning to cope with a mother with special needs by the age of twenty four. I felt I had been dished out just about all that life could throw at me — unfortunately life wasn't done with me just yet.

As I mentioned, my younger siblings were more dependent on my mother than I ever was. I assume this was due to the fact that for as long as I could remember I had spent only half my time with her. The other half of my time was spent with my grandparents, where I was given perspectives my siblings unfortunately were not. I was taught a different way of life, taught how to problem-solve, how to see the brighter side of life instead of the oftentimes negative, gloomy, self-defeating outlook my mother walked around with. It was through this that I decided at a rather young age which approach I wanted to take with my life, and this contributed to a lot of tension between my mother and me. While she wanted to constantly focus on the problems she was faced with, I was looking for solutions, a habit I wish to this day both my siblings would have adopted.

In the blink of an eye it could all be gone. What are you doing in-between the blinks?

—Author Unknown

With my mother not around, it left my sister and brother to pick up the pieces as well, and to an outcome that would lead to more tragedy in life. My sister, Ashlee, resorted to drugs and alcohol as a way to medicate the pain from the reality that our mother would never again be the mother she knew. Her choice to do so is one I struggle to understand to this day after witnessing all the heartache and pain it caused us during our childhood. This would be the beginning of Ashlee's downward spiral. It started with her giving up custodial rights of my niece, just a toddler at the time, to her father. She began living in a dangerous area of Detroit, where she took a job as a topless dancer at the local establishments. Despite all of my and my stepfather's efforts to intervene, she was not receptive. We just couldn't get through to her, no matter what approach we took.

I can recall one of the last holidays we spent together. It was Christmas and it had been around a year since I had seen my sister. We hadn't spoken due to a fight between us after I caught her stealing my mother's medications and I called her out on it. As they say, time heals all wounds however, and I felt compelled to try to make amends by inviting her to my house along with my parents for a family Christmas Eve dinner. At this point, my mom was using a wheelchair to get around and had regained a large part of her memory. I can remember being extremely nervous to see my sister. I was filled with anxiety over which version of my sister would show up that night. When she walked through my front door, her beauty struck me as it did with anyone who saw her, a trait that always shined through even at a young age. She had long smooth black hair that looked like silk draped over her shoulders. Her eyes were big and green, with long eyelashes surrounding them. She had a brilliant white smile that would light up a room and the sense of humor to go with it. When we were kids, we used to sit around watching comedy movies, and I would belly-laugh the entire time as she recited all the funniest lines of the movies verbatim. She could make you laugh with just her body movements, like something you would expect from Chris Farley, if she felt so compelled.

I couldn't recall the last time I saw that version of my sister, at least until she walked in my front door that cold winter night. I could immediately see it wasn't the usual version of my sister we had all grown accustomed to, the replacement even a complete stranger could tell was inebriated in some way, shape or form. No, this was the girl I grew up with, and I couldn't have asked for a better Christmas gift. The first few hours of the night went exceptionally well with all of us gathered around the dinner table enjoying a wonderful meal and reflecting on past times. Even though my mother suffered the injuries she did and would never again be who she once was, I remember looking around the table overwhelmed with joy from the thought of having my family back. Unfortunately, this was a feeling that would be short-lived. Shortly after finishing up dinner, Ashlee snuck away to the bathroom with a bottle of prescription medication she managed to take from my mother's purse when no one was looking. Within twenty-five minutes of her bathroom break, it was clear to all of us that she had gotten her hands on something, despite denying it when I asked her. I asked my stepfather to count out my mothers medication to confirm I wasn't going crazy. This angered my sister, just as it had so many times before, leaving she and I arguing back and forth. I was angry because she had ruined our night by making such a poor choice, and she was angry, I assume, because I had called her out on it. By this time, my sister had already made arrangements for a friend to pick her up, and before I knew it, she was out the door. This would prove to be the last time I would see my baby sister. Her addiction would continue to consume her for the years to come, continuing to push she and I further and further apart, to the point of no longer communicating.

Unfortunately this is not how the story ends. One Sunday evening while sitting with my wife and kids, I received news that my sister had passed away. It was my stepfather who originally got the news and immediately called to inform me. At this point, it was not clear to us how she had passed, all we knew was that her body was at a hospital in down town Detroit, where she had been living. My parents and I made the forty-five minute drive to the hospital that night to identify her body. I remember the feeling of being overwhelmed from confusion as to what actually happened to her and a deep sorrow from the thought of my sister being gone. I was also fearful of what I was about to witness at the hospital. How do you actually prepare for something like that?

Once we arrived at the hospital, we were directed down a hallway to a desk filled with busy nurses. After what seemed like only a moment, one of the nurses noticed us and asked how she could help. After telling her why we were there, she informed us that Ashlee was located in the room directly adjacent to the desk we were standing in front of, just a mere ten feet away. I remember turning around and staring at the door I was about to walk through, incapable of truly believing my sister's lifeless body was on the other side of it. We still had not learned what actually happened to her, if it was a drug overdose, a homicide or perhaps just natural causes, but beyond that door lay the answer, an answer I wasn't sure I was prepared for.

As the nurse stepped in front of us to open the door, I instantly felt my heart skip a beat because I knew that what I was about to witness was something I would never forget. The nurse stepped aside to allow us to enter the room. As I attempted to make my way into the room, I can still recall the feeling of my feet being extremely heavy, as if they were trapped in cement. My parents were in front of me and my younger brother ,Tyler, who had ended up meeting us at the hospital since he had been living a short distance away.

I can still hear the sound of my mothers cries as she was wheeled into the room and saw her daughter lying on the hospital bed. A white sheet covered her from the shoulders down. Her long black hair was in shambles, and you could tell she had been crying from the smudged makeup and mascara trail running down her cheeks. The paramedics had left a device called a combitube in her mouth, which are a set of tubes placed down the throat to help someone breath during resuscitation. Even though I was standing in front of her cold lifeless body, it was still nearly impossible to believe this was my baby sister lying in the bed in front of me.

After just a few moments, a representative from the hospital came into the room to discuss what they knew about how she had died. I was crushed to learn that at the age of twenty-six, Ashlee had decided to take her own life by strangulation. A fate I still to this day struggle to understand. The report read that she was found in the attic of a small, rundown duplex she was living in. She had apparently suffered a foot injury weeks prior that left her forced to use crutches to get around, which would have made it extremely challenging to even get up into an attic. This shows just how desperate she was to take away her pain. In the days following, it was my responsibility to collect Ashlee's personal belongings from her home.

I had made arrangements to take my younger brother with me, not only for assistance but also because he had spent some time living with Ashlee and knew exactly where she lived. Tyler had been battling his own addiction issues since my mother's stroke and often retreated to my sister during those times. Having never been to my sister's home, I was shocked to see the conditions she was living in, as we got closer to her home. It was an area of the city that reflected something you would see in a movie. Filled with old, rundown homes that had either been abandoned or partially burned down. There were dilapidated buildings and signs of poverty on every corner. She had been living on the upper level of a duplex, with a young family living below her. As my brother and I approached one of the two doors located on the front of the home, her neighbor stepped out of the other. She had seen us pull up and recognized Tyler. After saying hello to him, she asked who I was, and Tyler quickly replied, "This is our big brother," a nickname he had labeled me with when we were just little children. She seemed a bit puzzled at first when looking at me, and later stated I wasn't what she expected. She assumed that with how troubled Ashlee was and the similarities in my brother's lifestyle choices, it would only make sense that I would share the same hobbies. After initial introductions, I asked her if she could tell me anything about my sister's life leading up to her death. She quickly mentioned how she and Ashlee had become good friends easily, which was no surprise to me knowing how charming she could be. One of the stories she told me was how Ashlee struggled on a daily basis, often not even having the means to feed herself. She expressed that even though she had children and very limited resources, she would let my sister eat dinner with them a few nights out of the week to try to help. This was a very difficult story to hear, and even now, years later as I sit and type this in a local coffee shop, I struggle to contain my emotions.

After making our way upstairs into Ashlee's home, I was dumbfounded by what I saw. The house was virtually empty and poorly kept up. The carpet had stains throughout it, and there were holes in the walls from what looked to be a person's fist. The windows were so dirty that you could barely see out of them, and the house reeked with odor. There was a couch in the living room that looked as though it was found on the side of the road, and a small, outdated TV that didn't work was sitting on the floor. Next to the television was the mirror portion of a large vanity propped up against the wall. Her friend said Ashlee often would sit on the floor in front of it and do her makeup before she headed out. As she told me this story, I noticed a message she must have written just before she made her trip up those stairs into the attic. It was written in her red lipstick on the mirror, and told how she was tired and could no longer carry on. As we continued to make our way through the rest of her home, it was clear that aside from a mattress located in her room on the floor, a few dishes and a few pieces of silverware that she owned nothing else. The exception was a brown cardboard box her friend directed us to that was hidden under some clothes in her closet. She said this box contained my sister's most valuable possessions. She knew this because Ashlee would pull it out almost daily to go through it. To say that I was anxious to see what filled this box would be an understatement! I assumed I was going to find something like her favorite pieces jewelry or perhaps some nail polishes, but I didn't. I found a box filled with photos and memorabilia from our childhood. Photos of our family, my mother, my stepfather, me and my brother, as well as photos of her five-year-old daughter she left behind. I remember almost falling to my knees while looking around this place my sister called home, looking down at an old tattered cardboard box, thinking of how awful my baby sister's final months of life must have been. How lonely and helpless she must have felt in her final moments.

It is during our darkest moments that we must focus to see the light.

—Aristotle Onassis

As much as I would like to say this is the last example of traumatic experiences I have had to deal with, I would be lying if I did. I would yet again be forced to endure more personal loss. Six years after losing Ashlee, I would suffer the loss of my brother Tyler.

Tyler was the youngest of the three of us and easily the most energetic of the bunch. It's my opinion that out of all of us, he got the least amount of attention growing up. Looking back on it, I am certain it was largely due to my mother's inability to adjust to the extra needs he required. At a young age, he was diagnosed with attention deficit disorder with hyperactivity. Anyone who has a child who shares this diagnosis knows firsthand the special set of parenting skills you need above and beyond what's considered the norm. Our mother simply did not have the capacity to offer him what he needed. As I mentioned earlier, she was faced with her own set of mental illnesses to cope with. This, coupled with the fact that my stepfather worked around the clock as a car salesman to provide us a life far greater than anything we had experienced in the past, made his ability to offer any extra support to Tyler virtually impossible. Now add in the mix that half my time was spent with my grandparents, it didn't leave Tyler with the support he needed in the younger years of his life, the years when most of us are learning how to deal with our emotions and problem-solve. And in these less-than-favorable circumstances, Tyler grew up as all children do, and eventually added the diagnosis of bipolar disorder to his list of obstacles.

Despite this, he was always happy and easygoing when we were kids. I remember being shocked by his ability to just brush off getting the third degree when he got in trouble, which he often did. I probably found this difficult to understand because I was without question the most sensitive of the three. There was a six-year age difference between Tyler and myself, which often made it challenging for us to share similar interests as we were growing up, but we still stayed close, as all brothers do. As I mentioned earlier, it wasn't until my mother's stroke that things started to spiral out of control for both my siblings. Tyler resorted to drugs. Based on what he told me, he starting with alcohol and then marijuana, and at some point graduated to heroin, which has proved to be a current epidemic in the youth of our local communities today.

After starting his heroin habit, he began stealing from people, including my parents, to support his habit. Our mother was an easy target for him because she was impaired, and by this time, incapable of thinking for herself. He would just say he was coming to visit, and she was none the wiser. As I said, my stepfather was at work most of the time, and Tyler knew where he kept his rainy-day fund. Despite the loss of Ashlee, when I found out about my brother's behavior, I felt I needed to distance myself from him. I found myself yet again shocked and confused by Tyler's choices and the lifestyle he was living. The lifestyle he knew caused us so much pain growing up. The lifestyle that took our sister from us far too early. For the next few years, I no longer communicated with him, with the exception of rare occasions. This was very difficult for me because he was my only sibling left at this point. It just seemed that no matter what I said or did to try to help him, he would inevitably do the opposite.

Tyler's choices eventually began to catch up with him in the form of legal trouble, and he was arrested a number of times. With each time leading to a longer sentencing, it forced him to sober up. This turned out to be one of the best things that could have happened to him. In the beginning, when he would become incarcerated, it would force him to sober up, like I said, but unfortunately, he wasn't locked up long enough for a real transformation to take place. Before long he would be released and back out on the streets. With his criminal resume growing and his prison visits extended, it not only forced him to stay sober longer, but in the process re-evaluate some of his thinking.

It was around this time that I began to receive letters from my little brother, filled with a side of him I assumed I would never see again. I would write him back and eventually began talking on the phone with him once a week. For the first time, he was upbeat and positive about turning his life around, asking me questions he had never asked before. Questions like, "How do I open my first bank account?" or "What's the first step you think I should take to try to get a job when I get out of here?" It was in these conversations that I felt like God had finally given me a chance to be the big brother Tyler always referred to me as. I felt like it was a chance to help my little brother in ways I had never helped my little sister. Tyler and I went to work on a plan for what he needed to do once he was released.

By this stage in my life, I was a busy husband and father to four amazing children. The time not spent with them was juggled between taking the steps necessary to reach milestones in my career (this book being an example) and focusing on the success of our business. To make the statement my brother's track record was slightly tarnished would be a huge understatement, and I knew this. I knew I had the safety and well-being of my family to consider, but after some discussions with my wife, I decided I would offer Tyler the chance to come live with us. As already mentioned, I felt compelled to step out of my comfort zone with Tyler and do what I thought would truly help him after losing Ashlee like I did.

You could imagine his excitement when I made him the offer. An offer that was contingent on only a few things. The offer was I would buy his food and he could stay in my home rent-free as long as he stayed clean, held a steady job, and helped around the house with what ever was needed. There was also one other rule I made no exception for: He was allowed no contact in any way with his longtime on-again/

off-girlfriend. I knew she was an addict and a bad influence. He had told me story after story of how he knew he would always risk relapsing if he was ever put in compromising situation by her, and he feared she would do just that. I knew if I could just keep him sober and them separated long enough, he could turn things around for himself. After discussing, he agreed to my terms and moved in upon his release from prison.

The following months would prove to be some of the most amazing times I would share with my brother. We would often just sit and talk about life, about our childhood and all that we had endured. It was a time in my life that was filled with experiences and emotions I was desperate for after losing Ashlee. To have Tyler safe under my roof and under my guidance, to not have to wonder if he was OK or if he was on the streets somewhere hoping for just a small piece of food to put in his belly like my sister did was a feeling of relief I will never forget. Part of our plan was to get Tyler on his feet and teach him the skills he needed to function like a normal human being, and we went to work on that plan immediately. Luckily he was able to line up a job working with one of his past sponsors (a person who agreed to mentor him through his recovery process from addiction) as soon as he was released. This allowed us to move to the next step on his list, which was to get him set up with his first bank account at the local credit union. Naturally a close second to that was to get him established at the local gym with his first membership. I mean, priorities are priorities, right?

Despite the fact that I was extremely busy raising four kids, running a business, chasing my own dreams and making sure my wife wasn't neglected along the way, I can still remember such a deeply gratifying feeling from being a part of these experiences with my brother. Even though he was a grown man who should have accomplished these simple tasks years before, I was grateful to finally be the big brother he needed. I was never given the opportunities for the normal experiences most take for granted with their siblings. I had never even been in a car my brother was driving because he had never had a license, let alone a form of transportation other than a bike or skateboard.

This next experience Tyler and I shared is an odd one to try to explain. Even though I had spent countless hours in gyms and was always one of the more in-shape individuals in the those gyms, even though I could perform at a significantly higher level than most and was complimented wherever I went, I was never able to share these accomplishments with the people I truly wanted to impress. Don't get me wrong, I am flattered every time someone pays me a compliment on my physical appearance or how strong I am, but when you're a young boy, it's always your dream to impress your mom, dad, brother or sister. I had never been given this opportunity until now. Even though we were both grown men at this stage of our lives, to see him look at me in astonishment and filled with excitement as if he were partnered up with Arnold Schwarzenegger as I took him through workouts with me was a special experience. To have him say how proud he was of all of my accomplishments inside and outside the gym and how I motivated him to want to do better, to do his best, is a personal achievement that I'm not sure I'll ever surpass.

Unfortunately my newfound relationship with my brother

would be short-lived. Despite all my efforts, Tyler eventually broke the one rule I had no exceptions for by starting a relationship with his ex-girlfriend. As I knew it would, this spelled disaster, and he quickly picked up the old lifestyle that she came with. I knew all too well what was next with his need to fill a rapidly growing addiction, so I was left no other choice but to ask him to leave my home. Tyler's life after that was filled with a lot of the same struggles our sister was faced with. As was the case with Ashlee, my stepfather and I lost contact with Tyler despite all our attempts to keep tabs on him. This was followed up with yet another call I had hoped I would never again receive.

It was a Thursday evening around 5 p.m., and I was at work, as I usually am. I was in the middle of training a small group of clients when my cellphone rang. It has always been my professional opinion that it is rude to answer my phone when I am training a client because they have paid for that hour with me and deserve my utmost attention. So when I heard it ringing, I let the call go to voicemail, as I always do. I did happen to glance down at it while it was ringing though, and took note that it was "Pops" calling, the name I've always kept my stepdad filed under in my phone. I assumed he was calling just to shoot the breeze and tell me about how his day had gone, as he often did, so I figured I would give him a quick call back between clients.

Two minutes later, my cellphone is ringing again, and now it is my wife. Again, I don't answer because I know if there is an immediate issue, she always follows up with a text message. Immediately after my cellphone stops ringing, the front-desk phone rings at our fitness center. At this point, my clients are on a short break, so I run over to check the caller ID on the phone — it's my wife now trying to reach me on another phone. At this point it is clear something is wrong, so I immediately pick up the phone. After my usual "hey what's, up I'm with clients," she replies "Dean," which instantly causes my stomach to hit the floor; she never calls me Dean unless I'm in trouble or something is wrong. She follows it up by reluctantly telling me my stepfather had called her when he couldn't reach me and informed her that Tyler had passed away.

I remember for the first split second thinking he had to be wrong! There was no way possible I was going to have to bury another sibling. There was no way I was going to have to say goodbye to my last sibling and be left an only child. I quickly closed up shop and rushed to my parents' house, where I found my mother hysterical from the idea she had lost yet another child. After taking some time to comforting my mother, I pulled my stepdad into another room to ask for details on what had happened to Tyler and how he found out. He explained that Tyler might not actually be gone. It might actually be a mistake. He had received a call from one of our childhood neighbors. She told him that she had received word that Tyler was missing and there was an unidentified body in the morgue that matched his description. My stomach instantly dropped at the thought of having to yet again go identify a body, but what choice did I have? I wasn't about to have my stepdad go through something like that again all alone. I also felt compelled to go to ensure that if it was my brother, he was taken care of properly.

My stepfather and I decided that just the two of us would go the following morning. The body was at a morgue in downtown Detroit that neither myself nor my stepfather were familiar with. To be honest, I'm not sure I know many people who are actually familiar with places like that. I cleared my schedule that Friday and was at my parents' house by 8 a.m. My stepfather asked me to stop at a local gas station before we left town so he could grab a coffee. As I sat waiting for him to go in to get his coffee from the Tim Hortons that was attached to the gas station, I started to play out how this experience was going to go based on what had taken place with my sister. I found myself feeling overwhelmed by how the process was going to go and quickly realized I had no idea what to expect because we were going to a morgue, not a hospital like in the case of my sister.

I also found myself thinking about what costs were going to be involved. I knew my parents didn't have the means to take care of my brother's final arrangements and that I would have to do my part financially. It was during this thought that a friend and fellow firefighter from the fire department popped into my head. I remembered him mentioning during the day he was the director of a large funeral home. I quickly pulled out my phone and called him to ask if he was familiar with where we were going and what I should plan to experience. I didn't even expect him to pick up the phone because it was first thing in the morning on a workday. Not only did he answer, but he just so happened to be off work that day. When I told him why I was calling, he immediately insisted I come pick him up so he could assist us in the process that was about to take place. He not only knew exactly where we had to go, but he even knew the exact people we needed to talk to. He also had all the expertise to handle the paperwork side, turning a potential nightmare into a quick and simple process. Despite initially feeling reluctant to take him up on his offer because I was certain he could find much more enjoyable things to do with his Friday, I knew I needed his help and we were just a mile down the road, so I took him up on his extremely kind gesture.

When we arrived at the morgue, we were asked to show identification and told we would be placed in a room with a television screen mounted on the wall. This screen displayed an image from a camera that was located in the room where they held the deceased. They explained they would make just the face visible on the screen, and at that point we would be asked to identify if it was in fact Tyler. I have to say I was somewhat relieved to know we weren't going to be placed in the same room with the body. Especially after finding out that this John Doe had been in the morgue for the better part of three weeks.

We were greeted by the investigator who was in charge of cases that included unidentified bodies, and were asked to follow him. He took us to a door located just a few feet away and asked us to step inside. As we walked into the room and I glanced up at the screen, I knew within seconds it was my little brother, despite the fact that he looked nothing like himself. It was hard to make out details due to the poor quality of the camera and the black-and-white coloring on the screen, but it looked as though he had been in a fight due to what looked to be bruising and lacerations to his face. The investigator read the report stating Tyler had been found deceased in an abandoned house located in a very poor area of Detroit. The house was known to be used by drug addicts as a place to get high. The investigator stated that he had more than likely died from a drug overdose. When I asked about the blemishes I saw on his face, he stated that it was from blood pooling due to that fact that when he passed away, he was facedown and wasn't found for some time. At this point the toxicology report was not complete, but it was later confirmed that he had gotten his hands on a bad batch of heroin laced with fentinol. My little brother had turned twenty-nine just days before his death, leaving behind two young daughters.

The days following were spent making my brother's final arrangements with the help of my colleague from the fire department. I felt it was my responsibility to step in and do this, not only to take some pressure off my parents, but I also felt deep down that Tyler would have wanted his big brother to make sure he made it to his final resting place safe and sound. With the help of my friend, I was able to do just that. I was allowed to accompany Tyler on his final journey to the crematory. I was able to be with him and say my final goodbyes as they loaded him into the cremation chamber. Although it wasn't an experience I would want anyone to go through, I was grateful to be by my brother's side for his final step.

To tell you that any of this was an easy experience would be a lie. I will say this section of the book has been the hardest to write, without question, because none of this was something I originally intended to include in this book. Up to this point, not many people knew these stories because I don't prefer to share them. I did not choose to add them for sympathy from you or to depress you, for that matter. Nor did I include them to try to prove that I have had it harder than you, or anyone else, for that matter. I am sure some of you have suffered events more tragic than the ones I described. The reason I decided to include these personal stories about my past is to best illustrate a significant purpose of this book's existence: to illustrate the fact that each and every one of you who picked up this book is capable of the highest levels of success regardless of circumstance.

I am a normal human being, just like all the other fitness professionals you see on social media or on the cover of your favorite magazine. I have kids and all the responsibilities that come with them. I have a marriage to tend to and make sure I am putting the necessary time and energy into. I have a business with a long list of clients to make sure I take care of and provide the best service possible to. And as you now know, I have experienced struggles, heartaches and pain. I could easily have thrown in the towel after any one of these events and told myself it just wasn't meant to be. If only I wasn't born into such a tragedy-stricken family, I could have achieved my goals. I could have done something great with my life. I could have written a book or helped hundreds of people to achieve the unachievable. If I had allowed any of these situations to take control of me, to stress me out or worry me, then I am in fact throwing in the towel and giving up on myself. That's not to say that I don't catch myself at moments feeling overwhelmed, concerned or unsure, but I have programmed myself to ask one simple question every time: "Will my choice to stress or worry about this situation solve it or make it any better?" Would stressing or worrying have brought my sister or brother back to me? Will stress or worry miraculously undo the trauma to my mother's brain, allowing her to walk and talk again? As we all know, the answer to each of these questions is no, absolutely not! The difference in why you're able to provide that answer so quickly and effortlessly in regard to my challenges or struggles but not your own is simply the emotions you do not attach to them! After all, they're my problems, not yours. You see despite that fact that I hope all of you reading agree that the personal stories I shared with you are tragic and sad, despite this, they still don't have the same effect they would if it was your mother who'd suffered a stroke or your sister who'd committed suicide or your brother who'd overdosed. The stories don't affect you in a way that makes you want to skip your workout tomorrow or go grab a tub of ice cream out of the freezer and force-feed yourself the entire gallon in hopes of making yourself feel better. The reason why is because you're not directly impacted by it and therefore don't attach excessive amounts of emotion to it. If this were your brother, your sister or your mother, there is a high probability that your workout would be skipped and that ice cream would get eaten. This is why it is so crucial you teach yourself to become aware of your programmed responses. Is skipping your workout going to fix what's stressing you out or worrying you? Is consuming a giant tub of ice cream going to make things better? Nope! It's always interesting when I hear clients or members who find themselves overwhelmed from stress tell me how they couldn't bring themselves to work out due to their stress levels. Little do they realize that their physical capabilities to carry out that workout they chose to skip were not hindered in the least bit. The body does what the mind tells it, and the sooner you realize this fact, the better off you are. The sooner you realize that stress and worry are not tangible things that grab a hold of you or that can be injected into you, they are manifested in the mind and therefore always under your control, the better. You choose whether you're going to be stressed, worried, happy or sad — and the list goes on.

Once you fully commit to this way of thinking, a beautiful thing happens. The ball is placed back in your court. You make the rules and you're in charge! In the case of the unfortunate happenings in my past — yes, I was deeply saddened by them, I was absolutely confused, frustrated and disappointed, but I quickly reminded myself I could literally do nothing with any of these negative feelings. I recognized they served no purpose whatsoever and had the potential to destroy me if I made the choice to hold onto them. If I did hold onto them, I could very well end up sharing the same fate of my siblings or, as a best case scenario, I never would have aspired to do what I was put here for, I never would have pushed myself to achieve what I am fully capable of, and I would have given up my opportunity to help and serve others. Stop giving up your own opportunities; stop giving up on what you're already so capable of!

Let's walk through the information needed to ensure that you're fully aware of just how toxic and counterproductive stress and worry can be for you physiologically. Reacting to situations in an overly stressful manner will create a long list of physiological issues. I want to touch on just a few that will create huge hurdles along your fitness journey if you allow them to.

The first one is an increase in your cortisol levels, which will essentially cause your body to hold onto excess fat primarily in the midsection area. If you are looking to shrink down your midsection, this is an obvious issue. If you currently are a person who tends to react to situations in a stressful or generally negative manner and you find yourself struggling to make physical changes, especially related to your midsection, this type of reaction on your part will make changes to this specific area of your body difficult and could very well be a driving force behind how that area of your body became problematic in the first place.

The second hurdle you will most definitely be challenged with in relation to stress and worry is your body's global response to it. Your body views internal stress no differently than external stress. An example of internal stress would be to become stressed out because you're running late, or perhaps you're dealing with fussy children and your patience has run out. Perhaps you took a promotion at work and the added responsibilities are more then you bargained for, or there are the all-to-common marital challenges so many are faced with. In other words, I'm talking about stress that is in your head or self-manifested.

Now for external examples, these would be related to actual physical injury or trauma. You accidentally trip over an abandoned toy left at the top of the stairs, sending you to the bottom a lot quicker than you had originally planned, leaving you with a sprain or fracture of some kind. Or perhaps it's our favorite time of the year, when all our children go back to school only to come home with every imaginable illness you can think of in the first week, which we inevitably end up contracting.

Your body doesn't differentiate between the two types of stress I just described and therefore responds to both with the same safety mechanism. It's an automated response that is hardwired into your nervous system called the-fight-

or-flight response. In this mode, your body's main focus or intent is to protect the operating systems that sustain life while shutting down all other less-important normal functions of the body. Operating in this condition is not only an unhealthy way of living, but it, without question, stops you in your tracks to attaining that new and improved version of you. In the rare cases I've seen clients continue pushing themselves, still applying all the necessary tools despite high levels of stress, it slows their progress to a snail's pace, at best.

If you didn't already catch the irony of this chapter here it is. If you stopped ten woman on your local streets and asked each of them to name off the top of their head the ten most stressful endeavors they can think of, every single one of those women would include trying to lose weight or attempting to improve the physical appearance of her body in some way as something that is highly challenging and highly stressful. Interesting how one of the more stressful things a woman claims to experience in life is mitigated by removing stress from the equation. This helps to outline why so many women fail long before they ever even start.

As I mentioned, I am not a self-help expert or positivity guru, and I am not here to go into detail on how to better cope with stress, but I will tell you the light at the end of the tunnel is as you improve your overall health through starting your journey, you will note drastic improvements of your overall state of mind or moods, and will therefore manage stress in a more effective way. I have a long list of clients who will attest to this improvement. What most people struggle to realize because the change is so gradual is that as we let our overall level of health fall from the top of the mountain down toward the valley of illness, disease, aches, pains and premature aging, our body becomes less and less capable of coping with normal stresses we all face every day. We start to view what was once a small problem with a simple fix as a colossal problem that holds the capability to end our world as we know it. Again we don't recognize this change in our response or how we view that same problem because it takes us years to fall down the metaphorical mountain. The sooner you plant your feet firmly on that mountainside, grab a hold of the rocks in front of you and start your journey back to the top, the sooner you will witness firsthand how quickly your inabilities to cope are reversed with every inch you pull yourself up. It is the initial climb where I see most give up though, and it is without question the hardest part of the journey. The trick is to simply look at the mountainside standing right in front of you. Don't create unnecessary stress or discomfort by standing at the bottom of the mountain while looking up to try to figure out how far the top really is, or how long it's going to take to get there, or all the risks involved if you fail and fall back down. Reach up and grab a hold of what's in front of you. It's useless to look any higher than what's actually within your reach. Take your time and work your way up with each new rock you grab a hold of, and always remember that every mountain has a top, so as long as your consistently reaching the next rock, eventually you're going to hit the top. It's just a matter of time.

A great example I use to teach my new clients how to grab the rock right in front of them rather than reaching too high is to simply commit to thirty days of staying dedicated to the practices and principles in this book. If you do, I promise you will find yourself in the same position virtually all my clients do. You will have climbed your way out of the valley and high enough up the mountain that those same stresses that seemed so unbearable, that seemed impossible to overcome and stopped you in your tracks, are now minute at best. You'll find you're so high up the mountainside that you don't even recognize them as stressors any longer. Now they just blend into the rest of the beautiful view from above. This is the pivotal point that I work tirelessly to get each woman I work with to, because I know this is when the real magic starts to happen.

I will walk by faith even when I can not see.
—2 Corinthians 5:7

TESTIMONIAL

Dean Mitchell has changed my life in a way I never imagined. Not only am I in better shape at 47, than I have ever been in my whole life but after joining Dean's facility a year ago I am still seeing changes everyday. Dean has given me all the tools I need to be a healthier, better me! He is so dedicated to helping each individual make the changes they want to see. It's almost impossible to fail!

I described walking into Mitchell Fitness Solutions to a few of my lady friends that wanted to join after seeing my results... you walk in and it's like going shopping for a new body. Dean will make it happen. All you have to do is the work!

I remember when I joined my first thought was... I won't have time to get to the gym, to prepare my meals, to be in social setting and keep making changes. WRONG!!!! So wrong...it has become part of my everyday life! I don't know how I was ever able to raise my family and work full time without Dean and his principles in my life. I am strong, filled with energy and feel amazing! It's not something you need to make time for, it just becomes a part of your everyday life. Without it I could never accomplish what I do in a day!

Thank you Dean Mitchell for changing my life. Not only has he helped me achieve my goals but he has given me the tools to rebuild me from the inside out! He is not only my teacher but my dear friend. He is a blessing to so many people who have made the change.

It's impossible to fail with Dean... The only way to fail is if you don't want it. Even for those that walk in wanting just a little change, the results are so unbelievable that 9 out 10 take it to a new level! Dean and his fitness program have not only changed my life, but in the process he has given me a whole new meaning for friendship and family with the other girls in the program! We support each other and we push each other to be the best that we can be. Dean Mitchell you are my Angel on so many levels!!!

My friends and family can't believe the changes I've made since starting Dean's program. My kids are so proud of me and my jeans love me too... Lol. Dean Mitchell has a gift for customizing a plan that works for YOU. He is dedicated to make the changes you want to see. The before and after pics speaks for themselves!

If I could give anyone a gift, it would be the Dean Mitchell experience! A gift for life! The only question you will ask yourself after starting the his program is.... How did I ever live without it! Give yourself that gift!

With Love and Gratitude Silvia

The influence of a mother in the lives of her children is beyond calculation.

—James E. Faust

4:

TURNING YOUR CHILDREN FROM A BURDEN TO YOUR BENEFIT

Nearly all of the females I work with are busy mothers desperately attempting to juggle a hectic life and all the responsibilities that come along with the title of mommy. It wasn't until I found myself working with an astounding number of females who were faced with this circumstance that I was forced to seek out effective methods of integrating what is paramount for each mother I work with to reach her goals while keeping up with the needs of her children. Although there is often a short adjustment period, each of my clients has found the information in this chapter to be extremely useful. In not all, but most cases, I initially find a natural disposition with those I work with to always want to put their children first. As much sense as this makes, I ask you to be careful when taking this position. The reasons are for other than what most of you are thinking. Bear with me for the next section of the chapter. I ask you to hear me out and have an open mind when reading this chapter of the book. I will remind you, I speak only from experience with a long list of highly successful female clients, and as I mentioned, I am a father of four little ones myself.

I am not saying, in any regard, that your child or children

should be neglected or mistreated. All I would like you to do is pay close attention to whether your actions are providing them with the things they need, or providing you with excuses as to why you cannot commit to the lifestyle changes needed to reach that new and improved version of yourself. There is a very important distinction between those two scenarios, so my advice is to take a moment right now and ask yourself the following question in regard to your child or children's needs: "Does this need require immediate attention, forcing me to drop everything, or do I have the ability to rearrange my schedule to fit both the need and the requirements of my fitness program?"

"Is my child's need for their pleasure (i.e., a trip to the mall, sleepover with friends) or does the need fill a requirement of their responsibilities (i.e., a trip to the library to research a homework assignment)."

"Is there an alternative resource (i.e., car pool, spouse, neighbor) I can use to tend to this specific need?"

"Is there an alternative resource (i.e., daycare, babysitter, spouse) I can use to tend to my own need?"

"Have I exhausted all options in finding a way to tend to this need without giving up my own?"

"Will my children's life be put in danger if I do not tend to this need?" This question is meant to sound a bit dramatic to wake you up to the reality that we as parents have the ability to overdramatize situations or needs when it comes to our precious little angels.

I would like to touch on the second question to ask yourself and show how it is a perfect example of how we often give up our own nonpleasure needs (i.e., requirements to reach your goals) so our children can have a little fun. This is not to say you shouldn't condone fun for your kids; I am simply saying it shouldn't be at the cost of achieving your own personal health goals, goals that add up to more time on this Earth with your children and children's children.

I implore you to be honest with yourself and the answers you come up with because this exercise is oftentimes challenging and can prove to be a tough pill to swallow. In most cases, you will be left facing the reality that the current excuses you've held on to so tightly are just that, excuses. I don't mean for that last sentence to sound obtuse, but having four kids of my own offers some personal experience as to how easy it can be to make excuses, to skip a workout or change up what should be on my menu for the day when the kids are thrown in the mix, and remember, I'm the professional.

Here is another exercise to try when establishing if you're truly being bogged down by your little ones. Sit down and write out a list of what you would be doing differently, both physically and nutritionally, to reach your fitness goals if you didn't have those little angels to spend all your time and energy on. Be sure not to limit the list at all. Examples could be attending your favorite aerobics class at the local fitness center in town. Or perhaps finally hiring yourself a personal trainer and getting started on a new program. Now I want you to add your little ones back into the equation and label what direct need you provide them with that takes away your ability to still participate in each activity listed. How do your little ones stop you from hitting that aerobics class or getting started with that personal trainer? Do they literally make it impossible or rather just inconvenient? I often find when my personal clients participate in this activity, they come to the conclusion that the biggest impact their kids have on them reaching their goals, is related to scheduling conflicts more than anything else. In other words, it's never an impossibility, but more likely, a matter of an inconvenience. Regardless of what you find to be true in your case, you now have your key qualifying questions to help you create solutions. Always remember when asking yourself any of the questions, you must answer with as little emotion as possible. Replace the usual emotion attached to your responses with rationale, and you'll always find a solution or way to make it all work. I know this sounds easier said than done, so I will use a past conversation with a client to paint a better picture.

Here is how the conversation went:

> **Me:** I noticed from your weekly check-in that you did not reach your weekly goal for your targeted cardio requirement. Is there anything I can do to help you?

> **Client:** No, no. It's not you, it's the kids. They have really been pushing my buttons this week. My son received a poor grade on an exam despite the effort we both put in on studying for it, and my daughter lost her

cellphone, which meant I had to make special trip to the cellphone store for a replacement, and oh, don't even get me started on how expensive and time-consuming that trip was! Ughhhh, this week has just been shot so far!

Now let's do a little comparison. If you can recall my first rule of having the proper mindset and the story told to illustrate it comparing you with two different version of the same painting. Why don't we apply that here, and see what we come up with?

In the case of you holding in your possession a cheap knockoff painting and your week turning out like the one my client had... The last thing on your mind would be tending to a worthless painting. You wouldn't devote any time to it or the requirements of owning it. Who cares? It's worthless! Why don't we compare the requirements I gave my client, such as the task of performing the necessary amount of targeted cardio needed to ensure the progress she's looking for in the mirror? Let's compare that, with the responsibilities of owning that cheap knockoff painting? Tasks like maintaining it properly and keeping it safe from being damaged. It makes total and complete sense why you or anyone else for that matter would have zero interest in taking the time to perform the necessary tasks the painting requires. After all, is it really that big of a deal? It's just a cheap knockoff, and you had an extremely stressful week filled with unexpected situations that you had no control over!

Now let's take that same week filled with all the stressful situations, filled with all the disappointment, filled with all the let-downs, and apply it to the case of the priceless painting. The one-of-a-kind painting to which no other painting compares. Priceless in value. It's the painting that everyone would love to have. Don't you think, that despite the unexpected week you were faced with, you surely would have made the time to ensure your painting was safe from harm? That no one tampered with it, that it was clean and maintained to the highest standard. Or, do you think you would have made the same decision you made with the worthless painting? The decision that the stress of the week is worth more than ensuring your priceless painting is safe and sound. I'm sure by now you're starting to see my point that there is nothing more effective then the right mindset. If my client who struggled and ultimately failed to meet her requirements that week reminded herself how truly unique and priceless she is, how she does in fact hold in her possession that priceless painting, she would have without question found a way to fulfill the requirement of her results!

For those of you who are reading this and saying to yourself, "I don't want to risk my relationship with my kids by taking some time and energy for myself," that is a completely justifying thought. I can say in the fifteen years of working closely with my clients, I have witnessed the profound effects that take place in the relationship these women have with their children as they move along their fitness journey. Initially they all share the same concern you do, that by spending time on themselves and striving to reach their fitness goals, they are taking time away from their children. Despite the fact that some of these concerns are related more directly to the age of your children, for the most part, unless the client is in the later stages of her life, this is a concern that finds its way to the surface. It makes total sense that if you're leaving your kids at home with a sitter or in the daycare so you can go work out you're clearly not present with them. Well that depends on how you define being present with your kids.

Odds are if you're reading this book, you're looking to change something about yourself physically, that at one point or another has bothered you. Perhaps its external flaws like cellulite on the back of your legs that keeps you out of what used to be your favorite pair of shorts or two-piece bathing suit in warmer months. Or maybe it's the size and shape of your arms that keeps you trapped in long sleeve shirts and sweaters regardless of the season you're in. Perhaps the changes you seek are internal. Maybe you're struggling with a low energy level that leaves you feeling tired and drained most of the day. Perhaps your immune system's ability to fight off illness has been reduced, leaving you sick half of the year. Regardless of which scenario you find yourself in, the bottom line is, you're mentally or physically affected in negative ways when your health and fitness are compromised.

How do you think those negative effects translate to your mood around your children? How well do you cope with being woken by a shrieking two-year-old in the middle of the night after already suffering from exhaustion long before you crawled into bed? Or, how well do you handle two children battling in the backseat of the car while on the way to school like two Roman gladiators dueling to the death, when you're coming down with the third cold of the month and all you can fantasize about is being dosed up on NyQuil cuddled up in between the silky sheets of your warm bed? What if simply taking a few hours a week for yourself translated to higher energy levels or a stronger immune system? What if just those few hours a week left you lighter on your feet while dusting off your pre-baby wardrobe? What kind of mood would you be left with if every morning you woke up feeling energized as if you had slept for a week straight, or if every time you looked in the mirror after your morning shower, you stood in amazement at the woman reflecting back at you? What kind of tone would that set for the rest of your day? I bet that mother or that version of you is one the kids would graciously take in trade for a few less hours of your time!

As discussed in the chapter covering worry and stress, we talked about some of the negative impacts they have from a physiological standpoint. Let's now talk about some of the huge benefits you can expect when applying fitness to your life on a consistent basis. Aside from the obvious facts that most people are already aware of, like strengthening your cardiovascular system or reducing your midsection, there are other improvements taking place behind the scenes. Virtually every internal process that takes place in your body on a daily basis is significantly impacted in a positive way. Your ability to cope with mental stress is dramatically improved. Think of exercise as another form of decompressing from emotional baggage you carry around. I have heard therapists tell their clients to scream into a pillow or possibly even punch it as hard as they can a few times. Performing this physical activity has been shown to help relieve the mental stress you've been carrying around with you. Exercise is another form of physical activity that has the same effect. Each and every one of my clients will attest to the fact that when they are left unable to exercise for an extended period of time it literally changes their overall mood and how well they cope with the normal day-to-day activities some would label as stressful.

When you exercise, your mood is naturally enhanced, not only through the decompression I just described, but also because as you exercise, you release feel-good endorphins that have the effect of leaving you in state of euphoria. Similar to the emotions you feel when you receive some really good news such as finally getting that promotion you've worked so hard for. The feelings of happiness, joy and bliss become the norm for you. You've all experienced this after you receive wonderful news, and you can pretty much guarantee that with the exception of a few circumstances, your day will turn out to be a great one no matter what happens moving forward. Imagine how effectively you could parent your child with feelings of extreme happiness on a daily basis. You have the power to achieve this anytime you want just through exercise. Maybe your intention is to reduce body fat and fit into your favorite jeans, or perhaps to finally be able to wear that two-piece bathing suit that's been neatly tucked away on some top shelf in your closet collecting dust since your first child was born. I can say with certainty that when you accomplish either of these goals, the fact that you can confidently strut around on the beach or finally purchase your favorite designer jeans is a huge milestone, but these accomplishments are only icing on the cake compared with the person you will have become on the inside!

Yes, your child can see you in that bathing suit and are excited by it without question, but not for the same reasons that excite you. They see you in your bathing suit or new pair of jeans, but they also see something else, something far more dramatic, far more exciting. They see the woman they call Mom who pushed herself past any limits she originally set for herself. They will see your success from all the time and effort you put into reaching your goals despite how tired you were. They see what the hours of cardio, the dedication to your fitness program and attention to the foods you eat have done for you. They see their mother's true potential shining through, and they know that with a willingness to not give up on themselves, they to can create any physical change or outcome they desire. They're excited by the lessons you have taught them along your journey. These are such invaluable lessons that they will take with them the rest of their lives! I have been lucky enough to witness this firsthand with my personal clients and their children, and these are by far some of the most moving experiences of my life. Watching young children grow into young adults and actually apply the principles they have been taught by their mother. Knowing they will never struggle with obesity, or have to take medication for hypertension or diabetes. Knowing their lives aren't at risk of being cut short from heart disease is a truly incredible thing to witness. By devoting just a fraction of your time and energy to yourself, I promise, in turn, you will be given the ability to show your kids the best version of you... a gift that every single one of us wants to be able to give our children!

TESTIMONIAL

I signed up with Dean to help me lose my baby weight from my pregnancy...I couldn't have done it with out his help. By the time my daughter was 6 months old I was leaner, lighter and felt amazing. You wouldn't be able to tell I just had a baby. During the program I felt amazing and had endless energy. Dean helped to keep me motivated and stay on track. I am pregnant again and cant wait to have Dean help me again. Even though I have the tools to do it on my own, his drive and dedication to his work will keep me coming back for more help.

Thanks Dean!

Peace is the result of retraining your mind to process life as it is, rather than as you think it should be.

—Dr Wayne Dyer

5:
YOUR FIRST LOUSY DAY

Strange title for a chapter found in a book created to make bad days a distant memory, right? Once you get yourself started in a program and have decided to commit to the new and improved version of yourself, one of the first things you can count on is never having to deal with another bad day, right? Wrong! This is one of the bigger misconceptions I deal with when starting a new client in one of my programs, so listen closely to what I'm about to say. You're going to have bad days ahead of you. You're going to have days when you feel tired, irritated, disappointed, frustrated — and the list goes on. You're going to find yourself looking in the mirror thinking, "Wow, I haven't made one physical change I was hoping for!" I personally believe this is triggered by your natural desire to use only visual changes to gauge progress. As logical as this approach might seem, because clearly we all want to see those changes when we look in the mirror, you need to keep a couple of key rules in mind in relation to how your body works. I want you to set down this book for a moment and get yourself a pen and notepad. Take notes on this section because the following are foundational rules I apply with each and every one of the ladies I work with.

Rule No. 1

You cannot spot reduce! In other words, you cannot pick one part of your body and decide to lose unwanted body fat from only that specific area. Your body doesn't work that way. If you find that one area of your body is shrinking, I promise you that the rest is as well. The reason you will notice it in one area of your body first is because that area usually has less that needs to go. This is why most of my female clients will find that they start to lean out in their face and arms first. With that said, you also need to keep in mind this means that the biggest, most problematic areas of your body will always be the last to go! I am sure this is disappointing news to most of you, but this should also shed some light on how easy it is for some of you to throw in the towel before you've actually started the race! When you look in the mirror, it's only human nature to automatically direct your eyes right to the area you feel needs the most improvement, not knowing this will be the last to go. This experience is usually followed up with extreme disappointment, along with frustration and hopelessness. Stick with it, ladies! If you're following the principles found in this book, you're well on your way. I'll make you the same promise I make each of my clients: The changes are happening right before your eyes... you just can't see them yet! A tool my clients find extremely useful in regard to this particular situation is to have photos taken periodically. Unfortunately because you see yourself on a daily basis in all of your glory, it's easy to overlook the transformation that is taking place because it happens so gradually. Having pictures to reflect on gives you a much better perspective as to how much you really have changed.

Rule No. 2
Food is NOT what makes you fat! It is actually the reverse: The lack of food and or consistent eating is making you fat. Did you know that if you didn't change any of the current foods you're eating and just simply started eating more frequently,

you would see physical improvements in the mirror! Here is why: Unless you're intentionally manipulating your diet to put your body into very specific state of operation metabolically — a state that is literally impossible to get into accidentally, called ketosis — you're doing more harm than benefit by skipping meals. There is much more to it than the catch phrase that's grown extremely popular: calories in versus calories out.

It is my opinion that you should be more concerned with nutrient timing and making sure you're providing your body with the macronutrients it requires based on that time of day and what activities are or are not coming. Examples of macronutrients are proteins, fats, starch-based carbohydrates and fibrous carbs. An example of a common mistake I see far too many people make is using the idea that as long as they are picking healthy foods, then they are eating an overall healthy diet and will see the results in the mirror by doing so. Under this idea, someone's dinner plate might include the following: a protein (red meat, white meat or fish), a fibrous carbohydrate (broccoli, asparagus or green beans) and a healthy starch-based carbohydrate (sweet potato, brown rice, whole-wheat pasta). Now I won't disagree that compared with what some of your other choices could have been, this is an overall healthy dinner. However, in the event you're really trying to go after body fat, looking forward to seeing that leaner version of you when you wake up in the morning, you're going to be hard-pressed to see those changes and will be left disappointed. Here's why. Let's apply my principle of sticking to nutrient timing, sticking to the rule of only providing your body with exactly what it needs when it needs to that dinner plate described earlier. The majority of the plate makes sense for the time of day, let's say six o'clock in the evening. This is the time that most of you will be winding down your day. Sure, the kids probably need baths and lunches need to be prepared, but overall the amount of labor-intensive activities will be minimal at this stage in your day. Under these circumstances, both the protein and fibrous carbs you're about to consume will be utilized by your body in a positive way. You will, however, run into an issue in regard to that starch-based carbohydrate you're about to eat . To put it simply, because you are officially done with any highly intense physical activities for the day, your body has no use for that type of a carbohydrate. What happens next creates the byproduct that so many of you cringe at when looking in the mirror. After your body realizes it will not need to utilize that starch-based carbohydrate for high levels activities, it will go to Plan B, which is to store it away for a rainy day. In other words, it gets converted into unwanted body fat.

This same rule applies to sugar and how it relates to nutrient timing. If you find that you like to have your little nightly dose of a sweet treat, you've got a better chance of witnessing your toddler reshingle the roof than seeing a slimmer version of yourself in the mirror. This doesn't mean you can't have a delicious treat at night, you just need to make sure it's sugar-free. Items you will always find in my house that are sure to cure a sweet tooth are sugar-free Jell-O, sugar-free pudding and sugar-free whipped cream, just to name a few.

You can also make it a point to become savvier when preparing your meals. Alternative methods of preparing the same meals is a staple with every one of my clients, otherwise they quickly become bored. This spells disaster when it comes to nutrition. An example of this can be found in the case of an evening meal I might request in the form of a protein shake with all-natural peanut butter added to it. I teach my clients to take the same amount of protein powder necessary to make their shake and make a thick pancake batter out of it using a small amount of water. Placed in a hot skillet that's been sprayed with a nonstick spray, it will quickly cook up into a pancake, needing to be flipped only once during the cooking process. After cooking the pancake, my client will take the same amount of all-natural peanut butter required for their shake and spread it over the top of their warm pancake. To finish it off, I allow them to top it with sugar-free syrup and sugar-free whipped cream, both considered free foods as far as I am concerned. Now they have taken that same old boring shake and turned it into a delicious treat sure to satisfy your cravings, all while sticking to the specific macronutrients I originally requested. Ideas and options like this one can be found relatively easily on the Internet if you know what to look for. In this case you're looking to stay within your macronutrient requirements, if at all possible.

Now going back to nutrient timing and why it has benefited my clients far more than any system that asks you to simply restrict your total caloric intake for the day. This next tip will offer you visual changes in the mirror even if you never got up off the couch! Your body picks up on the frequency of your meals and dictates how much energy (fat) to hold onto for future use. In the event you're eating one, two or in most cases, even three meals a day, there is a high probability that your body is in what I call "starvation mode." Because of the infrequency of your meals, your body chooses to hold on to stored energy (fat) since it doesn't know when you will be eating your next meal again. Operating in this state makes even the most diligent efforts in the gym offer little to no changes in the mirror. I will say it again: "If you're starving your body by restricting calories or eating only a few meals daily, your body will hold onto stored energy (fat) at all costs!" This illustrates why my clients are shocked to see their pant sizes shrinking despite the fact I have doubled their calories for the day.

Taking that same concept, let's flip the habit of eating three or fewer times a day. Let's say you're eating every three to three and a half hours, like I request my clients do. Now you are consuming energy sources (food) consistently, and the opposite response takes place internally. Your body realizes it has no use for that stored energy (fat) because it has a consistent external supply of it, and immediately starts utilizing it! To illustrate the metabolic effect the principle of nutrient timing has on your metabolism, I want you to take a moment and picture a campfire. This campfire represents your metabolism. Obviously you want that fire to burn as bright as possible for as long as possible. The only way to ensure this happens is to continually throw logs on your campfire. The meals I am asking you to consume represent those logs. Don't let your fire go out! Make it a point to throw a log on it every three to three and half hours, and reap the rewards of a metabolism that would rival that of your children. Apply this principle, and your fire will continue to burn bright for years to come. This is how my clients see changes that last a lifetime, not just for swimsuit season.

TESTIMONIAL

On June 21, my brother Julian Borg and I met with Dean Mitchelll at Mitchell Fitness Solutions in Northville, MI. We took our first measurements and received our new meal plan and exercise regiment. I remember being nervous because dean said to "wear shorts" for the measurements... and I've never been a shorts type of girl.

Over the past decade or so of my life, each year brought probably 5 different diets or fitness "pushes." Being a teenage girl in our world meant starving yourself until the scale said you lost a few pounds. College brought new unhealthy eating and drinking habits—from late night study snacks to pizza after late night partying. On top of that, I started off 2016 with 6 months of traveling in Europe...drinking copious amounts of cider in British pubs, crafting my own perfect pint of Guinness in Dublin, and who can say no to unlimited gelato and pasta in Rome....? (the answer is no one, i don't care what you say Dean). The point is... it all added up.

Coming back from that trip, I realised I was sick of starting over and over. It was like a constant science experiment figuring out what diets and exercise worked and what didnt. Should I stop eating bread? what about counting macros, what was that about?? and spinning classes seemed trendy, right? with all of these constant fitness fads consuming the industry, I felt like it was easier to just enjoy my pizza and ignore the problem. Then, my aunt told me about her journey at MFS, and I started to watch Dean's videos on Youtube. Everything he said made a lot of sense and I found myself watching videos for hours. In one video, he claimed that his plan for his clients was so effective, that if you stayed committed and completed his program, you would never have to go through the process of losing weight again. You could do it right, one last time. That struck a personal chord with me. That week, I made an appointment with him, and I dragged Julian along.

Dean taught us some crucial lessons about health and fitness in the first 60 minutes we spent with him. He taught us about losing fat versus losing muscle, and how most people out there are literally starving their bodies and burning off their muscle mass in attempts to lose weight. He taught us things that I wish I knew 10+ years ago.. and he made everything perfectly simple.

Dean works day in and day out to make sure that he can help as many people as possible. It has been such a blessing to work with him and I know that Julian and I consider him family. The 15 weeks were hard—mentally and physically. However, I can honestly say I have never been committed to something for this long. Every morning when I woke up this summer I felt leaner, stronger, and even more dedicated. I knew what I had to do, and I did it without complaining. I once watched my someone eat BBQ chicken pizza (my favorite) on the weekend and I didn't want one bite because I knew it wouldn't get me closer to my goals. I even brought almonds and turkey jerky to the bar one night because I didn't want to skip a meal. I went on vacation to Washington D.C. and I stayed completely on track— packing food for the drive and working out in the hotel gym.

I have been searching for the recipe to success all along, but I finally figured out what it is: Commitment to yourself and your goals + a plan backed with knowledge + a supportive network + a strong desire to change.

I won't lie… coming back to school has been tough. I have not been progressing as rapidly as I did this summer. As a stress eater, I am still trying to figure out how to stick to my goals and pull those homework all nighters. I am still trying to figure out how to stick to my meal plan with hundreds of temptations and the college partying lifestyle constantly surrounding me. I haven't been perfect and I physically feel different than I did before school started. Regardless, I am sitting here typing this post while eating my hardboiled egg whites in the library and I did 60 minutes of targeted cardio at 7am this morning.

I got majorly off track during the holidays and winter break, but when I was able to kick myself back into motion, I knew exactly what I needed to buy at the grocery store and what meals I needed to prep to get back on track. That is what is so special about Dean's plan. It forms habits and lifestyles, not quick 30 day fixes. I know how to measure my meat and veggies, I know what to look for when I need a quick protein fix. I know how to maximize my time at the gym when I only have 30-45 minutes.

I wake up every morning and I remember how long it has been since I first walked in to Mitchell Fitness Solutions. I think about how lucky I am to have a healthy, strong body, and a mentor as amazing as Dean. I think about how far I have came in 15 weeks and I visualize what I could achieve in 15 more. I think about the hundreds of pounds of protein I have probably consumed, and the hours and hours I have spent in the gym. I don't even have to look in the mirror to know it was worth it and I am immediately reminded why I want to make today better than yesterday.

I can't wait to see how far these habits take me and my brother. I can't wait to mess up or fall down, because I know I have the tools and support system to get right back up. I can't wait to see what Dean accomplishes in the near future and watch how many more lives he touches. If you are looking to make a positive change in your life, check them out and give them a call. You won't regret it.

If you do what you've always done, you'll get what you've always gotten.

— *Tony Robbins*

6:
THE MAGIC INGREDIENT NEEDED FOR LONGTERM RESULTS

This next chapter is a big one, not only because of the amount of material that needs to be covered to properly educate you, but also because there is so much negative publicity and false information surrounding it.

This has by been by far my biggest hurdle to jump over with the females I work with, and I believe it's due to lack of proper education. Women tend to run for the hills when they hear the words "resistance training." A lot of what I discuss with my members and personal clients relates to the fact that at the end of the day, we are all made up of the same stuff. Take a moment to let that fact really sink in. It never fails that during an initial meeting with a new female client, I quickly pick up on the misguided ideal she has that, she needs to stay as far away from weights or resistance training as possible because she runs the risk of accidentally developing overly large muscles, the kind of muscles that take away from her feminine appearance. The conversation usually includes her making the statement, "I need to be careful so I don't end up looking like you!" After regaining the breath that was taken from my lungs after that metaphorical punch to my gut, and getting over the initial shock that she thinks what has taken me the better part of twenty years to accomplish with hours and hours dedicated to workouts, cardio and religious meal prep, can be achieved by her accidentally. I have to remind myself that this is a valid fear shared across the board by females, and I do understand it. With how popular the sport of competitive bodybuilding has become with females and how much information is at your fingertips, it's easy to see how you could be misled to believe you have the potential to achieve that look if you're not careful.

I will take the same approach in this book as I do with each of the ladies who work with me. Let's discuss what resistance training really does for the female body, and I will leave it to you to decide if you're going to include it in your overall fitness regimen.

If you haven't picked up on it by now, at this stage in my career my main focus is providing a woman with long-term results — not just immediate-gratification results, as I so affectionately call them. I do so through focusing on a number of different components that you can find throughout this book. One of the most crucial ingredients, or golden ticket, for not only achieving results but also ultimately sustaining them is to keep your metabolism moving as quickly as possible. Muscle is the driving force behind it; to make it as simple as possible, muscle equals a faster metabolism. In other words, muscle has a direct correlation to how fast your metabolism will move. It hopefully makes sense at this point to want to increase your daily metabolic rate as much as possible. I will let you in on how it's possible for the woman sitting at the table next to you at your favorite restaurant to polish off a half-pound of cheesecake with a bottle of wine and still look stunning in her dress. Here is how you to can get away with it. We have established that muscle has the ability to take your metabolism through the roof, but I am sure some of you are now fearful that in order to enjoy that piece of cheesecake and bottle of wine, you're going to have to end up looking like a distant cousin of Arnold Schwarzenegger. Pay close attention to this next part. Usually when I use the term "muscle," most woman think big and bulky like on a bodybuilder. This is not what I am referring to, and for the record, less than two percent of the female population even have the ability to build muscles to the size where they would be considered masculine in appearance.

OK, ladies, picture this for a moment. If I took two bottles that were exactly the same in size and shape, and I filled one of those bottles with fifty percent muscle and fifty percent fat, and then I took the other bottle and filled it with one-hundred percent muscle, leaving out the fat. Looking at the two bottles side by side, despite the fact that the contents are different, would the overall size and shape of the two water bottles still be the same? The answer is obviously yes. They are identical in outside appearance; it's only what's inside that is drastically different.

The point of this visual is to illustrate how you can still be the pant size 4, 6, 8 or 10 you are hoping to be regardless of the fact you're gaining lean, hard muscle. The effect that takes place in the female body through proper resistance training is to simply to fill those size 4, 6, 8 or 10 pants with nothing but lean, hard muscles. The stuff that doesn't jiggle. The lean, hard muscle that looks great in clothes — and even better out of clothes. The lean, hard muscle that, most important, drives your metabolism through the roof!

Let me take this one step further to ensure I really drive this principle home. Let's say I made an identical clone of you, and you're both identical from the outside with the same shape and size, but I created your clone with fifteen pounds more muscle mass on her body than you currently have. Again, let me remind you that you're both identical in shape and size; the only differences are internal. Now I take you both and place you each on the same piece of cardio equipment and have you both perform the same activity for the same intensity and duration of time. I can promise you that your clone will burn a significantly larger amount of calories, despite the fact that the activity and duration was identical. How can this be? Because her ability to burn calories is that much greater than yours. Hopefully this sheds some light on why, in woman especially, having muscles is a key ingredient needed for her success. This is, in my opinion, what separates my personal clients and their ability to maintain results compared with others who might have seen a reduction on the scale, but year after year struggle to maintain their success.

Now for those of you who don't already know, the main stimulant that promotes muscle growth is resistance training. The idea or intent behind resistance training is to promote or force a change in your body specific to lean, hard muscle. The change that can be expected in females is an overall leaner, firmer look, a reduction in unwanted jiggle, and being left looking exceptional in and out of your clothes. Now as I mentioned, traditionally you ladies think that when you apply resistance training, it means you inevitably will end up looking like Schwarzenegger with a wig on. This is, in fact, a genetic impossibility. Essentially because you do not possess the hormones required for your body to make those muscles so massive. These hormones are not included in a female's genetic makeup. In other words: You couldn't do it if you tried! Now for the ladies out there who are saying, "Well, I see these girls in magazines or on the Internet who are very big, very muscular and very masculine. How does that happen if what you're telling me is true?" Great question! In those cases, those woman are introducing exogenous hormones into their bodies to force those specific physical changes you see. They are looking for those physical changes and are working hard daily to promote them at all costs. They did not end up that way overnight because they stopped using three-pound dumbbells and opted for the five-pounders!

Now that we have established how it's not physically possible for you to look like Schwarzenegger, let's talk more in-depth about what you can expect from resistance training. I hear the request from a female in almost every consultation, so I am sure it's the same in your case. You want to get rid of the jiggle. The only way that's going to happen is if you pick up some weights. Muscle on the human body not only doesn't jiggle, but it looks great without clothes on top of it. Adipose tissue — or fat, on the other hand — will always jiggle and always offer a less-then-desired appearance when the clothes hit the floor. These are the facts, cut and dried. For some of you who can still fit into your size 6 or 4 jeans that you wore in high school but are saying, "I don't understand why I still fit into them, but I have more jiggle, and things definitely don't look the same as they once did, especially when I take them off!" The only difference is what is sitting inside the same size 4 or 6 pants that you're wearing.

And this brings me to another fact. This is a classic case I see far too often of staying the same size circumference-wise, but your body has lost the lean, hard muscle that it used to have from either lack of physical activity or starvation dieting, just to name two. It has since been replaced with fat, essentially leaving what you're made of drastically different. Refer back to the prior section of this chapter discussing the analogy of the bottles and what they are filled with. As I just mentioned, this change in what you're made of is often due to either one or the combination of lack of activity and lack of proper eating habits, forcing your body to go into what is called "catabolic state." In other words, your body seeks out alternative fuel sources because it is being starved, and it finds that alternative source of fuel in the form of your precious muscle. At this point, the replacement of muscle with fat has left you in a position that I've heard referred to as "skinny fat."

One of the bigger benefits a woman can expect from building lean, hard muscle mass that we have yet to discuss, is how your body gets stronger! Every female I have ever worked with loves this side effect because it drastically improves her quality of life. The majority of you reading this at some point in your life will become a mother, if you haven't already. In the event you don't have any of your own children yet, I will tell you firsthand life is so much easier with kids if you're physically stronger. I know it sounds silly, but how many of you struggle to carry a crying child with six other bags in your hand while trying to get your key in the front-door lock? To all you moms reading this, don't tell me you haven't been in this exact situation! Imagine if you had more upper body and core strength in a situation like that. For those ladies planning to give birth at some point in the future, I can't express how much of an upper hand you will give yourself during your whole experience, from conception to the birthing day, if your total body strength has been increased prior to taking that journey into motherhood.

Aside from the benefits listed above, there is one more I want to touch on that absolutely applies: the aging process. Your quality of life and risk for injury as you age will be drastically improved upon if you keep a steady resistance-training regimen part of your lifestyle. Have you ever experienced the devastation of an elderly loved one who takes a spill at home doing something as simple as getting up out of a chair or perhaps stepping down a small step? Aside from becoming a little more fragile, their muscles have lost the strength and ability to fire properly through lack of activity, making the simplest daily activities that you and I take for granted a real challenge and risk. The old saying, "If you don't use it, you lose it" absolutely applies here. It is no different than if you have perhaps suffered a broken bone or injury that left that part of your body weakened. When you attempt to use the part of your body that was immobilized while it healed, you can immediately pick up on the fact that something is off or not working properly, leaving you feeling weak and unstable. I have seen overall quality of life drastically improved in the clients I work with who are in the later years of life, from the grandmother who is able to chase her grandchildren around the yard in a fun-filled game of tag to the elderly woman who still enjoys dancing the night way with her husband. Resistance training, and fitness in general, is truly the fountain of youth guaranteed to allow you to stop your body's aging process and start counting birthdays backward.

TESTIMONIAL

I have paid many trainers in my past only to fall victim each time to doing the same cookie cutter, one size fits all routine. This is not the philosophy at Mitchell Fitness Solutions.

I met with Dean for the first time to discuss my fitness goals. I informed him of a neuro-muscular disease that I was diagnosed with that atrophies certain muscles in my body. Being somewhat of an unknown condition, he immediately researched it and came up with a plan of action. He began with a thorough assessment and evaluation of my physical and dietary situation. He then developed a program specific to my needs while being mindful of my limitations. Having one on one attention, in my case, was crucial. We have done a multitude of exercises and physical therapy and under his care, I have improved remarkably.

My diet, and knowledge of how my diet is working and why it is working, is paramount to my success. It also changes as needed. Since beginning with Dean in May, I have had 4 different diets. Each of them written specifically for me and adjusted as needed for evenings out and vacations. I am 43 years old and have never eaten better or felt better while dieting in my life. I have never wanted to stick to something and make a life change until now. We have all followed a diet before. We all have a pretty good grasp on what is healthy and what is not. Why I stuck to this one and not the others? I can only attribute my success and willingness to succeed to my faith and trust in him. He continues to educate himself on the latest and greatest studies. He makes himself the guinea pig, so to speak, before passing anything along to his clients. His positive attitude is inspiring. His exceptional knowledge and passion for his work is profound. He instills confidence and encouragement which makes you strive to be your best.

A friend of mine referred me to Dean and I can't thank her enough. My only regret is that I didn't find him sooner!

Listen to his podcasts. Read his book. Follow him on social media. You will be glad you did!

Real knowledge is to know the extent of ones ignorance.

—Confucius

7:
THE DREADED SCALE

Of all the chapters written in this book, my hope is for this one to resonate within each of you reading this for years to come. This is by far the most misunderstood topic I discuss with females. One of the primary reasons for so much confusion in regard to the all-mighty scale, I feel stems from so many of you being taught from a young age to focus on and worry about nothing other than that tiny little number that reflects back from the scale. This is a recipe for the instant-gratification results I touched on earlier that leave you with no chance for long-term success. This is the major driving force or reason behind why so many of you can never seem to maintain your results. I have written this chapter to explain exactly what the scale is in fact measuring, and how that measurement actually relates to your success.

Let me start with a question for you that I just touched on. What is the scale actually designed to measure? I ask this silly question not necessarily seeking your actual answer, but rather to get your mind to take a different perspective than the one you have used up to this point. So take just a moment to think about the question: What does the scale really measure? Assuming your answer is that it measures total body weight, you are correct, but did you catch the magic word? Did you catch the word "total" in your answer? If you didn't, "total" is meant to say it is measuring everything that you're made of. Keep that idea in mind as you continue reading this chapter because it is a key piece of information and will come into play shortly.

As most of you ladies know, the culprit of pant sizes climbing or being devastated when looking in the mirror as those pants hit the floor is the number on the scale going up. No news flash there, but I bring up this point to point out the crack in the foundation you have used to monitor your success up to this point. That crack in the foundation is this: The number one physical change women seek to make when they start in any of my programs is "to lose weight." They want to see that magic number on the scale drop every time they step on it.

So here is the problem and ultimately why I ask all of my personal clients to stay off the scale, unless I am in need of that information to adjust something in their program. Muscle is three times more dense than fat, so if you're spending your precious time in the gym trying to speed up your metabolism by increasing the amount of muscle on your body, it only makes sense that the scale will reflect a higher number. As a trainer, this is actually an initial change I look for. Oftentimes, if the scale drops too quickly out of the gate, it is a sign that one of the puzzle pieces of your overall program is not fitting correctly and is costing you the precious muscle that is key for the metabolism we all seek.

The reason I ask clients to stay off the scale, however, is to keep them in the required positive mental state we discussed earlier. The scale is indefinitely an emotional trigger for virtually every single woman I work with early on, and therefore should be avoided at all costs. Despite the fact that I cover this material thoroughly with each and every woman I work with, I know the profound effect that little number has had on her for so long and the negative emotions that come with it. I know those emotions have the power to overturn any logic I attempt to fill her mind with in the early stages of my programs. I know that if I don't steer her clear of that pesky scale for at least the first four to six weeks, that number she sees has within it a potentially disastrous effect on her ability to stay on track and committed to her own success. The irony is, in the initial stages of my programs, I am hoping for the number on the scale to move minimally, at best. In the event she does take my advice and stays away from the scale for those initial four to six weeks, I do note a significant shift in emotions related to what number pops up on the scale's readout when she eventually does weigh herself. This is mainly in response to the facts that by the time four to six weeks has passed, the amount of inches she has lost in all areas of her body, coupled with her clothes fitting much looser, cannot be denied. After all, how could you possibly stay upset about the scale not reflecting a number you had expected it to be while looking in the mirror and being amazed by who you see reflecting back?

Another compelling reason I always ask my clients to stay off the scale, especially when using it for a bearing as to how they're truly progressing, is as follows. Let's start with that metabolism of yours that we've already touched on a time or two during our new journey together. Remembering that metabolism can be defined as how quickly you burn calories or, in other words, how much slack you can cut yourself nutritionally. By now it hopefully makes complete sense to want to increase your metabolism or daily metabolic rate as much as possible. Again, it equals your ability to get away with a night out on the town with your girlfriends, a night that is sure to include a nice dinner and some cocktails. With the metabolism I can help you create, you can go out and truly enjoy yourself knowing you're not going to suffer any ill side effects when you look in the mirror the next morning. You won't miss a beat!

Most of you reading this are never given the opportunity to acquire this magic metabolism I speak of due to two major factors: a lack of proper education and misguidance from an industry standpoint. Most of you have been using the old thought process of restricting calories in the kitchen while burning up as many as possible in the gym. Or as I describe it to my clients and members: You're overtrained and underfed! This recipe will leave you with a minimal amount of that lean, hard muscle that drives your metabolism and a large amount of unwanted body fat — you know, the kind that jiggles! This lean muscle that I speak of is the golden ticket that so many of you miss out on but are in desperate need of. This is the golden ticket I provide for each of the ladies I work with, which leaves them lean, sexy and confident year-round, free from jiggle and falling body parts. Regardless of what curveballs life throws their way, regardless of any change in circumstance, they maintain the highest level of success because they possess a metabolism that would rival anyone, from an Olympic athlete who consumes five-thousand calories a day just to maintain his or her body weight to a young, energetic child who can live on a diet consisting of mac-and-cheese, Skittles, and peanut-butter-and-jelly sandwiches and not gain a single pound of unwanted body fat. That was not an invitation to test either of those lifestyles, but hopefully you get my point.

So what other options do you have to track your progress now that you have perhaps destroyed your scale through a ritualistic celebration that would rival one seen on an episode of *National Geographic* that was sure to including yourself and your closest female friends all dancing around in a candlelit room, each armed with baseball bats and a bottle of wine? Each of you taking turns swinging your bats to connect with that scale in a manner that would rival the way Babe Ruth connected his bat to a ball. All in hopes of releasing the pent-up aggression created from years and years of letting that little scale dictate so many aspects of your life, a scale you now know was a useless tool from the beginning. Or possibly you simply threw it away, which is fine too.

A tool I would highly recommend for tracking true progress in place of the scale is one I have already touched on. When you are first starting your journey, I recommend having someone you trust to not criticize you, someone you feel comfortable with, to take photos of you to help track your progress. Obviously, for some of you ladies, the thought of wearing minimal clothing while getting your picture taken sounds about as fun as grocery shopping with thirty-five three-year-olds. Just keep in mind I am not asking you to do a full-blown photo shoot for the cover of *Vogue* magazine. These photos are meant for your eyes only and will prove to be useful tools later on down the road, I promise. The purpose of these photos is to help you stay positive about your progress.

Even I will attest to the reality that there are days when I simply don't feel overly excited when looking in the mirror. For whatever reason, I woke up that particular morning with a sixth sense for finding every flaw or less-than-flattering part of my body. As you can imagine, what quickly follows behind my full-body evaluation is a state of mind filled with frustration and self-doubt. When I catch myself falling into this negative state of mind, I have trained myself to notice this shift in my emotional state and behavior, and I immediately pull out my secret stash of old pictures taken of myself from prior to my career in the fitness industry. Doing so not only instantaneously snaps me out of the emotional trash can I woke up in, but even more important, having these photos to reflect on gives me a strong ability to see a true perspective of just how far I have really come.

As human beings, it is easy to see our progress in a distorted view, primarily because we see ourselves in all of our glory, day in and day out. Now, in regard to the female population, I will say without question that each of you has a keen ability to be your own worst critics. The ability each of you ladies are born with to see the flaws reflecting back at you still astounds me to this day. Since changes come gradually over time, this leaves the door open to doubt and discouragement along the way, especially when equipped with the abilities I just mentioned each of you seem to possess. That is unless you have a trusty set of photos to reflect on.

There is nothing better than receiving a text message or phone call from one of my clients when she's having a terrible morning. Informing me that she doesn't want to get out of bed to come work out because she's exhausted from a sleepless night due to a spouse whose snoring could be confused for a tornado siren. Or, she had the pleasure of waking in terror throughout the night thinking she found herself in a distant rainforest sleeping next to a silverback gorilla after her toddler made his way into her bed in the middle of the night. At that point I simply ask her to pull out those pictures she took months prior or, in some cases, years ago. The next text or phone call is always, "OK, OK. I get it. I'm on my way!" Aside from the reasons already described, it is always nice to be able to take a moment for reflection and look back to where you originally started once you reach your goals. This is a great way to keep the soul filled with gratitude!

On to another option for tracking your progress now that you won't be stepping on any scales anytime soon. This is a tool I use personally as well as with each of the women I work with. It is my opinion that the most important number to monitor regardless of your goals, age or gender is not your BMI, but rather your body composition. Your body composition is essentially a measurement of what your body is made of, fat versus muscle. Thinking back to the water bottle and what it was filled with, it is the same concept put into an exact measurement that you can track. Let me take a moment to illustrate this in more detail. Have any of you had that friend or acquaintance who loves to talk about how skinny she is and has always been? How she fits into the lower-size options at your favorite boutique? She probably loves to make sure you don't forget how low that number is that pops up when she steps on the scale.

For conversation purposes, let's say she weighs in at a whooping 110 pounds. As exceptional as you or she may consider this number to be, you both should be far more interested in what her body composition reflects… what that 110 pounds of her is actually made of. In this example, her body composition number reflects forty percent. This essentially means that despite her ability to fit into a size two or four in jeans or the fact that the number reflecting back when she steps on the scale is a mere 110 pounds, of that 110 pounds, forty percent of her is made up of unwanted body fat! You know, the stuff that jiggles and falls to the floor when the clothes come off. My last statement was not intended to sound intrusive, but this is the harsh reality that so many women I meet are faced with. So many of you are starving your bodies of calories to stay in smaller sizes only to ultimately set yourself up for severe disappointment down the road. Lets apply what I've taught you up to this point and see exactly what is going wrong and leaving you virtually helpless in your ability to see any positive physical changes.

Sticking with the case of the woman who is small in size but maintains a higher body composition, she carries around a large amount of body fat. By default, she also carries around a minimal amount of lean muscle. Without question, her metabolism is nonexistent due to maintaining such a low amount of lean muscle on her body. This is a prime example of how you leave yourself with no ability to metabolize anything that would be considered tasty or a treat and therefore start crash dieting, restricting your meals or removing them completely. This is a recipe for disaster and an illustration as to what most of you have been experiencing and, more importantly, why so many of you have adopted this idea that food is what makes you fat... therefore, staying away from it at all costs.

I bring this up to help you understand that with a healthy metabolism, it will not only be a breeze to maintain the body, size and shape you wish to have, if you stick to your program with an effort level of just eighty percent, you will find it actually becomes a chore to gain unwanted body fat. A case in point of this that some of you may have witnessed can be found in the following story.

You and your girlfriend are out to eat at your favorite local Italian restaurant. Upon being seated by the hostess, you can't help but notice the couple sitting at the table across from you. Assuming they are married by the rings you spot on both of them, you find yourself staring at the woman seated politely with her slender legs crossed in a brilliant white strapless dress that was tailored with precision to fit the perfect curves of her body. You assume they must be celebrating an anniversary or some other important life event after your eyes finally make their way to the man sitting across from her. You can tell he is slightly older by the distinguished features his face holds. Through your continued scanning, you can't help but notice that despite the fact he is dressed in a perfectly pleated pair of dress slacks and collared button-up shirt, he can't hide the fact that underneath all of it he possesses a body that would rival that of a Greek God You can't help but stare momentarily at the lines his muscular silhouette creates even through that loose-fitting button-up shirt.

After your concentration is broken by the waiter who magically appears in front of you to take your order, you quickly glance down at the menu to make your choice. While doing so, you can't help but wonder what the couple across from you will be ordering. You can't help but wonder what special set of skills they must possess to order any food from a restaurant like this? Feeling guilty, you order the healthiest option you can find, settling for a salad and being sure to ask the waiter to hold the croutons and cheese and keep the dressing on the side. After all, how could you actually order your favorite lasagna dish with a couple like that sitting across from you, a couple who surely ordered boiled chicken with a side of steamed broccoli with no butter? How could you sit across and indulge in that lasagna and risk embarrassment when the woman who reflects so many of the same physical attributes you wish you had spots you with a forkful of lasagna, full of the delicious noodles, cheese and meat sauce your favorite restaurant is known for.

After taking your highly modified order, which reflects none of the ingredients you came in for in the first place, the waiter takes your friend's order and swiftly moves to the table across from you. By now your friend has noticed your interest continuing to shift from her and the latest gossip to the two sitting across from you. She quickly leans in toward the center of the table to whisper, "Um, hello? I am pretty sure that's his wife sitting with him!" Your initial reply is a quiet snicker to ensure neither of them hear you and become curious. This is quickly followed by you explaining that you're not interested in dating the man across the way; you're just intrigued to find out what a couple like that — a couple who maintain such stunning bodies — actually eat to look the way they do. Now both you and your friend are engaged, and you each begin to comically take guesses as to what the waiter will be bringing to their table. Aside from a few crazy ideas, you both agree he will be bringing salads as a worst-case scenario, which leaves you feeling confident in your dinner choice.

Some time has now passed, including some laughs and

harmless joking, when the moment of truth arrives and you spot the waiter making his way toward you. The tray he gracefully balances on one hand as he weaves his way closer holds on it two large white bowls, each filled with crisp bright-green salad. You also spot two small saucers, surely filled with the dressing on the side, as you expected the couple would have ordered it. With your friend's back to the waiter, you confidently inform her that the waiter is about to drop off the couple's dinner, and you both were correct in your assumptions of what they would order. As a feeling of relief washes over both of you for making the same choice the couple did, you can't help but notice the waiter is angling in your direction. You can't help but notice he is looking right at you with a look of satisfaction, as if he has finally arrived with your food you've been so patiently waiting for. By the time you note that you may have been mistaken, the waiter has arrived at your table and is placing the salads you were certain were intended for the couple sitting across from you. Your friend asks with a smile on her face, "Did you forget we ordered before them? I may have had to say something to management if their salads had come out first!" You reply with, "Yeah, you're right — silly me," coupled with a smile of your own.

Almost as fast as you see the waiter disappear into the kitchen, he reappears with another tray, showing off his unique ability to move with extreme grace and speed through the busy restaurant all while balancing his tray full of delicious foods with just one hand. You immediately notice him taking the same particular path he did with his last tray of food. This can mean only one thing: He is carrying the order you and your friend have been waiting patiently to examine. Filled with excitement, you reach across the table to smack your friend on the arm, saying in what was intended to be a whisper but most certainly came out as if you just won the lottery: "Here it comes, here it comes!" All this while not realizing your dearest friend has just placed a fork filled with crisp vegetables in her mouth, which sends both fork and food flying from her mouth, almost hitting the table next to you! The couple you've been mesmerized by the majority of your night looks over at the two of you to see what all the commotion is. As you glance in their direction to offer a moment of eye contact and a smile, your friend is wiping half-chewed salad and other vegetables from her cheek while she offers the same smile, although hers is filled with little pieces of green lettuce throughout her teeth. The couple offers a puzzled smile back, clearly unsure of what just happened. Skipping any apology elicited by your actions, you lean in toward your girlfriend, who's still trying to remove lettuce pieces from her lap, to remind her to quit fooling around, the waiter is coming! Distracted by your friend, you were unable to spot what the waiter was carrying as he made his way to the couple's table.

With his back now to you and the tray angled just right, neither you, nor your girlfriend, can see what he's placing on their table. As the waiter unloads his tray, you can't help but notice that the seconds feel like minutes. With the feeling of time standing still, the desire is building inside you to explode from your seat and into a full-blown sprint directly toward the waiter across the restaurant as if you were an Olympic sprinter. In this daydream, after losing your heels as you gain speed that would rival Usain Bolt's, you envision flying headfirst in an effort to spear the waiter, sending him flying through the air as if he were standing between you and the designer purse of your dreams on Black Friday. After coming back to reality from your daydream, you realize the waiter has since left, and you're shocked by what has been delivered to the table across from you. Both you and your friend are so astonished that you assume it must have been a mistake! All until you see the couple you were sure would have a permanent picture in the dictionary next to the word "healthy" start to dig in. As you are eating that delicious salad you had no actual desire to order, the couple across from you is enjoying, yep, you guessed it, lasagna! After all, it's the house specialty!

Both you and your girlfriend can't help but stare at this point — you both filled with a combination of jealousy, amazement and a hint of rage. Unfortunately, the amazement initially found in both of you, takes a backseat to jealousy, and now even more rage as you watch each of them polish off a one-pound piece of lasagna and follow it up with two giant pieces of tiramisu that could sink the *Titanic!* You find yourself asking out loud, "How in the world can they do that?"

So how do they do that? How can they sit back and consume all your favorite foods in one sitting? Foods that have a tendency to cause you to gain unwanted body fat just by looking at them, let alone eating them. To put it simply: "They possess the golden ticket." They're able to get away with a night like this and not miss a beat by making sure their metabolism is always operating as fast as it possibly can! The first step is making sure that the metaphorical bottle we described earlier, is filled with as much lean muscle as possible at all times.

Hopefully by now you're asking, "How do I get my composition tested?" Any reputable fitness center should have someone on staff to administer a composition test. There are a number of ways to offer the test, and all of them should be virtually free or cost a minimal fee. That being said, each option has different levels of accuracy. The quickest and easiest way is through a device called a bioimpedance machine or analyzer. This will give you a general idea, but it can easily be thrown off by things such as water intake or exercise on the day you're being tested. I always recommend and use handheld calipers with all my clients and stick to a seven-point site test. This is highly accurate and relatively easy to do. When getting the test done, you should not only be given what your composition numbers are, but also how they relate to your goals in mind. This is your time to ask questions to ensure you understand where you stand physically.

Having this knowledge under your belt will only add to your arsenal of tools to help you reach the highest levels of success. If you're considering working with a trainer, not only should they know how to administer this test but, more importantly, it should be included in any program you join with them. It is my opinion that this is the most important number to track when looking at true results and is also a necessary tool for your trainer to do his job. In the case of my clients, we retest every four weeks. This gives you a way to hold your trainer accountable for your results. After all, you're paying a lot of money for their guidance, shouldn't you have a way to track the results of all your hard work with something other than a pat on the back and a smile from your trainer?

TESTIMONIAL

I first met Dean Mitchell just about a year ago. Little did I know, that that day would now serve as the day, I would start to truly show up to my life!

My fitness journey thus far had been anything but easy! Like most, I was busy being somebody's wife, somebody's mother, somebody's daughter, employee and friend, but never just SOMEBODY! Just three years ago, I was 74lbs heavier and miserable! I avoided family pictures, functions and sporting events, because I was either too tired, too embarrassed of myself, or both! Additionally, I was facing some challenging health conditions, which by all accords, would only exasperate my then current state of poor health! I felt hopeless and total despair!

As you can imagine, the self-awakening was empowering, but there was such a long road to go and I didn't know the first thing about how to begin! I just knew what the scale said and it never spoke nicely! I jumped in with both feet! I joined a gym and sometimes worked out for three plus hours a day, sometimes twice a day! I ate protein bars and drank protein shakes and lived on 1000 calories a day! With this type of routine, I did in fact lose weight quickly! I lost over 9 pant sizes and 74lbs in 5 months! Everyone was praising me for how quickly I lost it and how great I looked! The high was awesome, until it wasn't! The excitement died down and the attention lessoned and there I was eating protein bars, limping into the gym, holding my continuous injured shoulder, still exhausted, still missing my children's life events, too tired to attend! It's funny, I had achieved what I thought I set out to do, the scale said wonderful things to me, so why was I still feeling the way I did?! I was still so very broken, maybe even more than before! I was tired of being tired, I was tired of being broken and I was tired of living my life in the hamster wheel!

On a friend's recommendation, I limped into Mitchell Fitness Solutions, holding my shoulder, desperate for an end to this dysfunction! Dean took all my measurements and performed an assessment, unlike one I had ever had before! His findings were shocking! Not only was I a much higher body fat percentage than I thought, but my muscle damage and overuse was extensive! My posture and form was something to be desired and my nutrition was near starvation! I was officially one big mess! He quickly put me on a program starting back to basics and carefully constructed a nutritional plan for me that almost doubled my calories. Following his lead, I showed up to training and followed his program. Within weeks, my injuries were healed and body fat percentage was dropping quickly! I was baffled! I was eating more, training less and my energy soared!

Since joining Mitchell Fitness Solutions, I've learned to work smarter not harder, that less is sometimes more and that great things happen when you get out of your own way! Dean understands that wellness comes from a mental place! His love, encouragement and words of affirmations, coupled with extensive knowledge are second to none in the industry! Thanks to him, I am in better shape at age 44 than I was at 18!

I wholeheartedly recommend Dean Mitchell!

Sincerely,

Kathy

Aim for the moon. If you miss, you may hit a star.

—W. Clement Stone

8:

WHY MY CLIENTS COULDN'T CARE LESS HOW MANY CALORIES THEY'RE BURNING

I want to start off this next chapter with a question: How many of you have that friend whose exercise regimen consists of cardio followed up with more cardio, and if she's feeling a little crazy, she adds in, yep, you guessed it, more cardio? Or perhaps this is you? If so, read closely, because this chapter covers what is, in my experience, the most common mistake made in the gym today.

Assuming you do in fact have a friend or perhaps someone you've seen in your local gym who fits this description, pay close attention as I teach you exactly why the choice to develop a fitness regimen that includes solely cardio and more cardio will prove to be a fatal error sure to kill any opportunity for that rock star you're so capable of becoming to smile back at you in the mirror. The habitual desire to do tremendous amounts of high-intensity cardio is most often found in women. I am sure this fact is a byproduct of men possessing an overly predominant "lazy" gene. No news flash there, right ladies? Oftentimes, when I do stumble upon a woman who fits this M.O; she indefinitely has an almost ritualistic approach to her cardio. While working in big-box clubs during past employment, I witnessed this unique but common approach to cardio time and time again. Despite the opportunity to select from more than one-hundred different cardio machines, this particular type of woman would choose the same cardio piece day in and day out. She has her one special piece of equipment that she uses every single time. She takes the same carefully calculated steps every time she begins her preparation for the event that is about to take place. The special placement of her towel, folded and draped over a particular section of the machine in the exact same way every time. This is followed by the careful and well-thought-out placement of her water bottle and iPod or iPad.

I find that indefinitely these individuals have two goals, two critical requirements, in mind to consider their daily dose of cardio a success. When she is executing her cardio, she must achieve these two key elements or she will surely feel she has wasted her time completely! The first of the two goals is to work at the highest intensity level possible. She does this to magnify her results and ensure she burns the maximum amount of calories possible with every stride and each tick of the clock. The second goal she is intending to reach is to go for the longest amount of time possible to ensure that her total amount of calories burned equates to the highest amount possible, often going as far as to compete with herself, striving to increase her total each time. Because it is crucially important that you understand what I just attempted to explain, I will abbreviate and recap the scenario: She goes as fast as possible for as long as possible to burn the greatest amount of calories possible! If by chance this sounds like your current habits, I sincerely hope you don't mistake my efforts to be as descriptive as possible in my storytelling to sound intrusive in any regard.

I commend each of the women who find this story familiar because it takes extreme dedication and determination to maintain the level of commitment I am referring to. My hope is to persuade you to utilize the tremendous work ethic you already occupy to your full advantage. Odds are if you invested in this book, you're hoping to find something that is missing. Something that has kept you from the success you seek. This book has that "something" and, more specifically, this chapter has the exact recipe needed when performing cardio to ensure your body is targeting that undesirable body fat when seeking out an energy source or, as we have labeled it up to this point, when your body is looking for calories to burn.

If you have ever been guilty of working at extremely high-intensity levels while performing cardio and committed to it for any length of time longer than a week, I'll bet you noticed that despite your efforts, you never were able to see the major physical changes you felt all your hard work and dedication elicited. Or, in the event you do not fall into this category, but can recall a fellow member at your local fitness center who you have witnessed nearly kill herself daily while on that piece of cardio equipment and its the same outcome. You've witnessed that member maintain a relentless work ethic for years, and which would put Mohammed Ali in the hospital, and they never seem to change. They still carry around with them all the unwanted inches they started with. Their body is still holding onto that same shape and size that they battle daily to change.

So what exactly is going wrong? For the purposes of the book, let's assume we are speaking of a female. How can it be that the harder she works in the gym, it still doesn't add up to more-dramatic changes in the mirror, to an accelerated rate of speed to the finish line? She's got the hard work and dedication, which is all she needs, right? Wrong! It is this idea that sets so many of you down the wrong path right from the start. To put it in the simplest form: The intensity level she is choosing to work at during cardio is far too high in relation to the physical changes she is desperate to see in the mirror, and here is why...

There are two major benefits you can expect from performing cardio on a consistent basis: *cardiovascular benefits* and *fat-loss benefits*. This is not to say that there aren't individuals out there doing cardio to help strengthen their hearts and lungs, but in all honesty, with more than a decade of training females, I can't recall when asking one of them what their goals are did I ever receive the response, "Oh I'm not doing this to get rid of any unwanted body fat. I really just want to strengthen my heart and lungs." Again there is a list of self-explanatory benefits if, in fact, this is your main goal, including increased life expectancy. I am candidly stating that this goal is rarely number one on the list. If as a side effect the client does improve her cardiovascular efficiency, she is undoubtedly happy to hear it, but again, I have always found the main focus with the female masses is ridding their bodies of as much of that unsightly body fat as possible.

Now that we have established the two main benefits of cardio, if your personal goal falls into more external changes than internal ones, the rest of this chapter will prove to be very valuable to you. As stated earlier, the majority of my clients are female, and virtually all of them, prior to attaining my services, use the total number of calories burned to gauge how effective they were during any given cardio session, and rightfully so. After all, the more calories she burns, the more fat she loses, right? Wrong!

You need to be more interested in what you're burning, not how much. My usual question I have for a new client or member who has just told me with a look of extreme excitement that she had burned 800 calories earlier that day during her cardio session. Being conscientious to not deflate her level of excitement, my response is always, "Wow! That's an outstanding effort. Can I ask you what you burned?" After an initial pause in her response as her eyes go crossed, the usual response I get is, "Well, obviously, fat." She couldn't be further from the truth! In fact, if she were correct, this book more than likely would have never been written, everyone would look amazing, and I would be unemployed. So what is going on then? Let's look at it through a different lens. I have attempted to structure the following information as delicately as I can to ensure I educate you while at the same time don't lose you through an information-overload coma.

During both rest and activity, your body utilizes energy to perform internal and external activities. Examples of automated activities would be tasks we aren't even aware we are performing at any given time, such as breathing or the continual growth of your hair and nails. There are also nonautomated activities our body utilizes energy to perform, such as swimming laps in a pool or running on a treadmill. Without a constant energy source of some kind, your body would not be capable of performing any of these tasks, and you would ultimately cease to exist. Now here is where things get a little more complex and we begin our decent down the proverbial rabbit hole so many of you end up lost in. Your body picks and chooses different energy sources based on what level of intensity or heart rate you're training at during cardio, or any other activity, for that matter. Whether you're sprinting up a mountain or lying in bed watching your favorite reality show, your heart rate during those times is dictating the energy source your body will pull from. That said, your next question should be, "What are those intensity levels (heart rates) and how does my body respond in each of them?" Great question! They are as follows, so grab that handy notepad you've hopefully been using up to this point and let the ink fly, because you don't want to be confused by this section of the chapter.

If you have ever heard the term "zone training" thrown around your local gym or latest fitness magazine, this concept is one I have used for years with my personal clients. I have found some flaws or discrepancies in the usual method most would define as zone training, and therefore have made some of my own modifications that have proved to be highly effective thus far. Let me illustrate it for you now. Assume that you possess a big beautiful home. In this home, there are a total of five rooms. In each of these rooms resides the same exact piece of cardio equipment. I will leave it to you to create in your mind whatever that piece of cardio equipment would be. Despite the fact that each room houses the same piece of cardio equipment, this is the only thing each room has in common with the other. Outside this, your cardio rooms become unique, and here is why: When performing cardio in any of the five rooms, you note a different feeling internally. While performing cardio in any of the first three rooms, your experience is, for the most part, a relaxed one. You feel as though you could do cardio all day long in these first three rooms. You notice as you move from the first room into the next, and finally make your way into the third of five rooms, your heart rate does seem to increase slightly but never reaches a point high enough to cause you to lose your breath. Even with your heart rate elevating slightly higher in each of the first three rooms, you find that while doing your cardio, you would be able to carry on a conversation with ease if someone asked you to, and at no point would you have even broken a sweat!

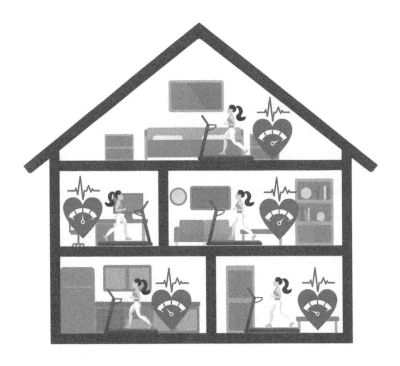

At least not until you venture out of the third room and into the forth. You immediately note upon starting cardio in that forth room your heart rate spikes to a much higher level. You're now working at an intensity level that is so high, it forces your breathing to become labored. You also quickly begin to perspire. Even though you would be able to still talk in the event someone stepped into the room with you, it wouldn't be without having to stop midsentence to take a breath. Now with just one room left in which to attempt cardio, you finally make your way from the fourth room of your house and into that fifth and final room. Upon beginning your cardio, you can't help but feel your heart rate spike to a level so high that if you kept going at the level of intensity demanded while in the fifth room, you would risk passing out! You can feel the pounding of your heart as if it were trying to burst from your chest. Your perspiration has increased to the point of dripping from your brow as if you were sitting in a sauna. With a heart rate this high, it would be physically impossible for you to spit out anything greater then a single word at a time due to the constant need to gasp for air. Keeping the illustration of your house, and the five cardio rooms in it, let's take things a step further.

Lets apply this concept to your five rooms: In my descriptions of each room, I am attempting to describe the fact that while you're doing cardio in any of your five rooms, you will indefinitely experience a different heart rate or intensity level. Apply what I taught you just a few moments ago in regard to how your body picks and chooses energy sources depending on the level of heart rate you're in at any given time, the level of intensity you're working at during any activity. Here is where your pen and notepad should become very useful! Ninety nine percent of the women I work with had been picking the wrong room to perform their cardio in, and here is why...

They have been taught to believe they should always burn as many calories as possible during cardio. Making the connection that a high heart rate or level of intensity while doing cardio equals a high amount of total calories burned, they work at all costs to make sure they do just that. If you found them in your metaphorical house, it would indefinitely be in the fourth or fifth rooms. Remember these are the rooms that requiring the highest heart rates or level of intensity. Therein lies the problem. As I mentioned before, it's not about how many calories you're burning, it's about what you're burning. Most would automatically steer clear of the first three cardio rooms in your house due to the fact that the heart rate while performing cardio in them is relatively low, meaning you're not going to burn calories at a very high rate. What if I told you that the main source of energy your body will seek to use while doing your cardio in rooms one through three will come from body fat? In other words, despite the fact that you might not burn as many total calories when in these rooms, all the calories you do burn will come directly from that pesky unflattering body fat! This obviously means if you are a woman who seeks to really target body fat while doing your cardio, you would be wise to perform your cardio in one of the first three rooms in your house. Let's cover some other key information in relation to cardio and the five cardio rooms of your house.

Everyone has what is called an anaerobic threshold (AT) that is based around your heart rate. Think of this AT as the threshold you cross over when moving from the third room of your house and into the fourth. If you make the choice to cross that threshold and move into that fourth room that demands a higher heart rate or intensity level, your body stops seeking out that unwanted body fat and looks for a new source of energy in its place. Or in other words, you're essentially asking your body to stop burning body fat and start looking for that alternative fuel source, which just happens to be glucose and your precious muscle!

Dean Mitchell

In the event you find yourself carrying excessive amounts of unwanted body fat and struggle to see any physical changes in the mirror no matter how much cardio you do, this is due to the fact that up to this point, you've been choosing the wrong room to perform your cardio in! Remember, anytime you choose to step over that threshold, or your AT, and move into rooms four and five, you are no longer burning fat; it makes total and complete sense why you and so many others never seem to lose that stubborn body fat. It has nothing to do with your fat deciding to hang around just to spite you or the idea that you were born with some rare genetic disposition that leaves you doomed to carry higher amounts of body fat for the rest of your days, it's simply that the conversation you're having with your body is the wrong one. Stop choosing the fourth and fifth room. Stop trying to burn as many calories possible. Stop telling your body to seek alternative energy sources other than the body fat you're so desperate to lose.

Despite the fact that these numbers will not be as precise as the ones my clients receive from me since I am not able to work with each of you personally, I have developed a formula that will unquestionably put you in the right room. This formula will get you in the fat-burning ballpark and on the fast track to finally reaping the rewards of all your precious time spent on that treadmill or elliptical. In relation to heart rate, as a general rule of thumb, I keep every single one of my clients below 135 bpm (beats per minute) anytime they step foot onto a piece of cardio equipment to do targeted cardio. When using the term "targeted cardio," I am saying that this is your optimal room where you will not only be asking your body to use body fat as it's main source of fuel, but also burn as many calories from body fat as possible. This is the cardio that is intended to focus exclusively on ridding the body of stubborn body fat and a foundational tool each of my clients uses to create and maintain any physical changes they wish to see.

I want to point out one other key issue related to performing cardio at a high rate or intensity level that is too high: Do you recall the energy sources I mentioned your body will seek out in the event you move above your AT, or from rooms one through three and into rooms four and five? If you remembered they were glucose and muscle, give yourself a pat on the back for being such an attentive student! Aside from the obvious fact that you're not burning off the body fat you thought you were when occupying room four or five, have you connected the dots of yet another detrimental problem? The peremptory side effect of utilizing muscle as a source of fuel is you're burning up the driving force behind your metabolism. If you remember from past chapters that muscle equals metabolism, then it should make sense that a loss in muscle is, in turn, a loss in the speed of your metabolism. You're essentially throwing that golden ticket right down the toilet! The same golden ticket I work tirelessly to provide every single one of my personal clients with, because it is the foundation to any physical transformation and, more important, the ability to maintain it. This is in fact the ultimate oversight that has kept you from the success already within your reach. This a mistake you cannot afford to make any longer!

If not addressed, you will suffer the fate of so many women I have met over the years but never had the opportunity to support. The women who feel helpless and depressed day after day because of a few elementary mistakes that have left them with a metabolism that wouldn't offer her the ability to smell a cookie let alone eat one. This, coupled with the fact that after years and years of utilizing her precious muscle as a fuel source, she is left with virtually none. Remember, this is the stuff that doesn't jiggle or fall to the floor when her clothing comes off. This is the stuff that makes her look so good in a bathing suit, the stuff that provides that priceless golden ticket she uses to spend frequent nights out on the town with her girlfriends drinking and eating her favorite foods without feeling guilty. This is the fate that too many of you face and ultimately why you feel like you're destined to walk around in a body you can't stand the sight of because no matter how hard you seem to work, nothing changes. I have the flashlight needed to guide you out of the darkness you have spent far too long in and into the light that has always been within arms' reach. This book is that light. Take grasp of it and begin to find your way out of the cold darkness that currently surrounds you.

I will warn you based on experience and feedback from clients, choosing to step out of that fourth and fifth room and move into one of the first three can be a bit of a challenge at first. Making the adjustment to slow yourself down and stop watching the calorie readout on the machine can be extremely challenging and downright nerve-racking at first. I understand this completely. After all, I am asking you to work at half the intensity level you're capable of and, in turn, burn half the calories you're used to burning. If you place the same trust in me and the methods I have created as my clients have, I can assure you that the level of success you will see will be like nothing you've ever experienced before.

Another reason the adjustments I am asking you to make to your cardio might test your willpower is mainly because most of us are creatures of habit. The ways we do things are usually developed for specific reasons, and the emotional connection we tie to them can often prove to be much stronger than initially expected. You might find your mood thrown off during the initial stages of implementing these changes. Often past clients have voiced feelings of being uncomfortable or in a generally tense, uneasy state. Keep your faith in the fact that the methods you've become so comfortable with haven't gotten you where you're trying to go. It's time for a new and improved strategy. You will face initial frustration when you see that total number of calories you've burned is substantially less than you're used to, but know that it is a step in the right direction.

I practice what I preach. For example, if you approached me in the gym after I completed an hour of cardio and asked, "How many calories did you burn?" I would smile and say, "I have no idea!" This is another example to help cement the idea of targeted cardio. If given the choice to do 45 minutes of cardio and burn a total of 800 calories with 200 coming directly from fat, or lower my intensity and only burn a total of 500 calories with 450 coming directly from fat, I will take the second option every day of the week. The big picture here is work less; burn more fat!

A few rules of thumb I use personally when I am attempting to ensure I stay in those first three rooms of the house — i.e., target my body fat or ask my body to seek out body fat as its main source of fuel — are as follows. I always make sure to work at a level of intensity that doesn't cause me to sweat profusely. At best I will barely break a sweat. Next, I always monitor my breathing making sure I maintain an intensity level low enough to ensure I am able to carry on a full conversation without any heavy or labored breathing between sentences. If you keep these two rules of thumb in mind while performing cardio, you can be sure you're in that fat-burning ballpark I mentioned earlier. You can be sure you've finally made your way into the right room of the house and are on your way to melting away those unwanted inches you felt you'd surely live out the rest of your days with.

To finish out this chapter, I will give you additional key information needed when designing your cardio program. When performing your targeted cardio, your duration should be a minimum of 20 minutes to a maximum of 60 minutes per cardio session. I define cardio to my clients as maintaining one consistent heart rate, or within five beats of it, for an extended period of time. As I mentioned, that extended period of time needs to be 20 minutes at a minimum. In the event you have been calling your daily dose of cardio a 5-minute brisk walk from your car to the office, I am sorry to burst your bubble. This is not considered cardio in my book. I would call that a warm-up. For those of you who like to do cardio for time periods longer than 60 minutes, the main concern and reason I don't recommend it for the females I work with is due to the fact that you run a high risk of burning up that your precious muscle — your golden ticket — after 60 minutes. The name of the game long-term is to always maintain your muscle and, in turn, you will always possess that golden ticket.

Since this chapter covers a ton of information, I would like to recap on the finer points. If you're doing cardio with the intention of reducing unwanted body fat, you must always maintain a heart rate lower than your AT. Or in other words, you should always choose one of the first three rooms of your house to perform cardio in. To a degree, this is oversimplifying a more in-depth conversation, but again, in the spirit of including only the facts you need to know in this book, this should always be your goal when performing targeted cardio. You're hopefully wondering by now how to find what your actual anaerobic threshold is. Here are some general guidelines that will put you in that fat-burning ballpark.

Age	Rooms 1-3 heart rate (within 5bpm or less)
25 or less	145 bpm
26 to 35	135 bpm
36 to 45	125 bpm
46 and up	120 bpm

Again, these numbers are not exact, but based on the data I've pulled from more than a decade working with female clients, these guidelines will provide you with the leaner, sexier version of you that you never expected to see reflecting back at you. In the event you would like more specifics, you can always seek out the guidance of a professional such as me, or perhaps another fitness professional in your area.

As far as frequency goes, or how often you should be doing cardio, here is a crash course on how I design for my own personal female clients the cardio portion of their program. Keep in mind the fact that done properly, targeted cardio is really the only tool you have in your arsenal that is designed to go after just the pesky body fat that has hung around far too long. One of the first key pieces of information I take into account when deciding the level of frequency I am going to ask that particular client to perform on a weekly basis is dependent greatly on her nutritional abilities. In other words, does she have the ability to do what I am asking her to do in the kitchen, to actually stick to the menu I have provided her with? Sure it's a nice thought to assume that every single one of you ladies reading this book just needs an effective diet placed in front of you and you will follow it to a T, but we all know this is simply not the case. There is always a learning curve when it comes to nutrition and a person's ability to follow through with what her dietary requirements are for her to achieve the success she is looking for. That's OK, though, and here is why. I ask the females I work with to give me only eighty percent perfection when following her diet or, in other words, eat the meals I ask eight out of ten times, no matter what her goals are. I find that most of you who I've never had the pleasure of working with have this big misconception that in order to achieve that leaner, harder, sexier version of you, it requires perfection in every aspect of what your doing one-hundred percent of the time. This is not true. In fact, I will tell you, with myself included, I have never met anyone who was perfect with every meal and every workout. We are all human and we all make mistakes, and here is how you get away with them.

My cardio and nutrition methods have a direct and strong correlation. They go hand in hand and can be mixed and matched to fit each individual's strong or weak points. When I am working with a female client, I know without question if she's falling off the nutritional bandwagon, but if her cardio is done perfectly and she's doing more of it than is required, she will get away with the mistakes she made in the kitchen and not miss a beat in the mirror. Vice versa, if I have a client who I cannot for the life of me get to do any substantial amount of cardio but her work ethic in the kitchen is absolutely impeccable, then the odds are she will likely continue toward the physical transformation she wishes to see in the mirror.

Now although in both of these cases she is continuing to progress and make the changes she is hoping for, those changes might be delayed slightly based on how far off she finds herself in any of the areas we have discussed. Remember the ideal situation is to commit to fitting all the pieces of the puzzle together, not just the ones you're naturally good at. To recap: If you find yourself struggling to make it happen in the kitchen, you'd better make sure you're pushing yourself to complete as much targeted cardio as possible to pick up the slack. The opposite obviously being if you find yourself falling behind on the cardio side, you'd better be willing to tighten up things in the kitchen.

This helps to illustrate what is by far the biggest error made by my clients over the years. You simply cannot afford a week that includes you falling apart in the kitchen and follow it up with zero targeted cardio or physical activity. This is a recipe for disaster that no one, including myself, can recover from. Going back to the original question asked, "How much cardio should I be doing?" hopefully you can answer that yourself by now. If not, keep this simple yet profound statement in mind: Targeted cardio equals fat burned, so if you're trying to tighten up things and get rid your body of the soft stuff, you should be doing as much as you are capable of while sticking to the guidelines listed above.

TESTIMONIAL

My journey started with Dean back in 2012. I was always a "big gym" kinda girl until I met the Dean Mitchell. Over the last several years I have trained with Dean, consulted with him on different eating plans and have come to genuinely care about him and his family as if I were part of it.

From a fitness perspective, he has pushed me to do more and eliminate the word "can't" from my vocabulary. Just a few months ago I decided once again to really get on track with my diet and "wow" what a transformation. Dean knew that he had to give me a plan that I could get my arms around and see results. He made sure to understand just how far he could push me and we worked through any obstacles. Dean's support, encouragement and reinforcement helped me to reach my goal and lose the weight and body fat I desired.

Dean is extremely knowledgable about his business and he juggle many balls to take care of his clients. I trust his recommendations and know that people see results if they follow his advice.

Thanks so much for making a difference in my life!

Debbie

Commit to the reality that your current habits have gotten you as far as you are today.

—Dean Mitchell (Author)

9:
EMOTIONAL TRIGGERS AND THE TRUE DEVASTATION THEY CAUSE

I personally believe we all have emotional triggers, and without question this has proved to be true in my clients. These findings have helped tremendously to shed some light on what I would consider one of the most overlooked issues with fitness-related programs or products to date. Let me start by clearly defining what an emotional trigger is so we are all on the same page. I would define it as any person, place or thing that you know has the ability to elicit a negative emotional response. Simple enough, right? Well, not quite. As simple as it is to define an emotional trigger, avoiding them is the challenge, but with focus, dedication and the knowledge you're gathering from this book, you will have the same success so many of my clients do. We will get into how to do this a little later in the chapter, but first I want to discuss with you how a subject related to your emotions has anything to do with shrinking that pesky midsection you've been carrying around with you.

Your emotions have everything to do with it, and it's my focus on them that has not only separated the methods in my program from so many others but, more important, proved to be the key ingredient in the recipe of success with the women I work with. If you were to approach me on the street and ask me to narrow down to just one reason why women fail when trying to achieve that new look, definitively my answer would be state of mind. At this point you might ask, "OK, fine. What's that got to do with my emotions?" Your emotions or the emotional state you are in is in fact the dictator of your mental state. No different from a taxi driver driving his taxi. That taxi (your mental state) is going to go wherever that taxi driver (your emotions) take it. I have watched more times then I can count a brand-new female client in my program who is highly motivated with the best of intentions crash and burn at the first sign of a struggle or a rock in the road. So what happened? Let's take a look together. Like I said, she was highly motivated and ready to rock-and-roll. What could have possibly happened to change such a positive position? Her state of mind changed. She's still physically the same girl who sat down committed, ready to go after her dream body. She is still made of all the same stuff, still has all the same physical capabilities she started with, but yet she's thrown in the towel before she really even got a chance to see what she was capable of.

This is a great example of what is the only thing that separates your struggle to see even moderate changes to that woman on the cover of your favorite magazine you wish you looked like. Please take a moment and let that last statement sink in — it has the ability to change your life like it has so many of my clients, if you let it. I will say it again just to help it really sink in: The only thing separating you from even the most out-of-reach goals you have is your state of mind or emotional state.

Unfortunately this is tough pill to swallow for a lot of women because it forces you to take ownership of where you're at physically today, in this moment. It forces you to deep down finally admit to the fact that if you want these changes bad enough, you will let no excuse stand in your way. My advice to you is the same I give each and every one of my clients: Use it. Use the idea that the only thing standing in the way of your success is the woman inside. If you take that advice, you will automatically regain control over yourself and your abilities. Control over the fact that if you want it bad enough, that woman you so desperately are searching for is already there; she's just waiting on you to change your ways, change your state of mind, change your emotional approach to the task in front of you. The ball is now back in your court. This is usually the step taken that forces the shift in my clients. It's a shift from being committed to the idea of reaching their goals but still clinging to that voice in the back of their mind reminding them they will likely fail, to being a woman who is no longer restrained by feelings of doubt or hopelessness, to a woman who is fully empowered and fully capable, needing nothing outside herself. She's driven by the fact that for the first time she knows her true potential and how limitless it is. The discovery of this missing link for so many women has blessed me with the opportunity to see some of the greatest transformations possible (both physically and mentally). This is when the real magic happens!

Now that we have made sense as to why these emotional triggers are such bad news, the next question is: How do you steer clear of all of them and finally make your own magic happen? Not to take a pessimistic approach or paint a contrary portrait in your mind, but you will need to be prepared to be diligent and consistent in learning this delicate dance. I have found for the woman I've worked with in the past that the most challenging part of the dance is being truthful with yourself in regard to what people, places or things are potential emotional triggers. This is difficult for so many because of the attachments that come with any one of them. After all, if you weren't attached to that emotional trigger — that person, place or thing that deep down causes you discomfort or pain, or causes a general state of negativity in your life — you would simply step away from it and continue moving forward.

In some cases, by just looking at things from this new perspective I have given you, it is possible that you will be able to identify and react differently to whatever your emotional triggers are and not need to attempt to eliminate whatever it is completely, but in the event that you find this step a challenge, this is the advice I give my personal clients that has proved to help. If you find you're struggling to pinpoint exactly what is causing you to feel stressed, depressed, anxious, fearful, tense, uncomfortable — the list can go on and on — I always ask my clients to simply take a step back and observe. More specifically, observe your surroundings and reactions to them as your normal day unfolds. Stay on high alert for any change in your mood or general disposition as you carry out your normal daily activities. As your day unfolds, you might find an emotional trigger to be a co-worker you often eat lunch with who you would consider a friend, but after observing her and her state of mind, you quickly realize the conversations or general tone of that lunch hour spent together is filled with negativity that only stirs your metaphorical emotional pot, leaving you with a less-than-favorable state of mind for the rest of the day.

Or perhaps it's something more direct, such as the mess left behind by your children, or possibly your spouse, on a daily basis that only adds more to your already overflowing plate of daily responsibilities as a mother and wife. Unaddressed these emotional triggers can leave anyone feeling overwhelmed and ultimately destroy even the most optimistic, especially during the beginning stages of entering this new chapter in your life. This is a problematic situation for a number of reasons. One I will highlight from past experiences with female clients is if you have a constant feeling of being overwhelmed by your normal day-to-day activities, if not addressed immediately, adding on this new endeavor or lifestyle can prove to be the straw that breaks the camel's back. Unfortunately, despite this overwhelmed state, often you will force yourself to start your health and fitness journey anyways, only you'll be destined to fail before you even get your feet firmly planted on the floor.

As they say, failure is not final, and I couldn't agree more with this statement. I am fairly sure by now I personally have failed more times than I have succeeded. The issue is not the actual fact that you failed your attempt at creating a better version of you, but rather the seed that has been planted under failing in those conditions. In that overwhelmed state, your natural disposition from a mental standpoint will be to simply accept this failed attempt as yet again evidence to the fact that you're destined to live out your days uncomfortable at the sight of yourself in the mirror, never again able to wear a two-piece bathing suit poolside or shop at your favorite stores for a new wardrobe. The reality of the situation is you could not be further from the truth though! You are not destined for any of those outcomes; you just need to do some simple rearranging or reallocating of your responsibilities outside your health and wellness so you're not left feeling so overwhelmed on a daily basis. Now for the million dollar question: "How do you give up important responsibilities?"

The biggest coward is a man who awakens a woman's love with no intention of loving her.

— Bob Marley

My suggestion if you have a spouse or are in a serious relationship is to begin with sitting that person down and asking for their support. If any of you find my strategy to be humorous or possibly fell out of your chair after reading it, I can assure you it wouldn't be the first time. I've gotten the same reaction from personal clients a time or two when discussing this crazy idea of asking a spouse or partner for their support. I've even become wise enough to make sure the woman I am having this comical discussion with isn't chewing gum so I'm not left giving her the Heimlich Maneuver in the middle of my office. Despite the fact that most of you find such a simple concept to be an outlandish and obscure practice, I want you to keep in mind that the author of this book is a man. In other words, the advice you're receiving is coming directly from the horse's mouth.

I neither claim to think like your husband or special someone, nor am I saying in the event that person does not share the same ideas I do that they are wrong and I am right. In an effort to ensure that the potential of finding death threats in my mailbox is minimal after the release of this book, I will simply share with you my perspective in regard to supporting someone I care deeply for.

A woman cannot change a man because she loves him, a man changes himself because he loves a woman.

—*Dean Mitchell (Author)*

It is my philosophy that through my commitment to another human being, whether it be the less-permanent pledge of dating exclusively or through wedding vows and the two magic words "I do," I am also committing my efforts and energy to the support of her success in all her endeavors. The efforts and energy I speak of should not be with conditions or prejudice. I should have a genuine interest in supporting all of her endeavors, not just the ones I find of value. Despite the reality that I might not always understand or agree with what my mate has set out to accomplish, that's OK because it's not my job to evaluate her choice or give her permission. A responsibility I do have is to recognize that in her decision to commit to whatever endeavor it might be it is a sign of how significantly important it is to her. Whether it be devoting her free time to learning ballroom dancing or, in the case of this book, she has set her sights on improving herself physically, her ability to achieve the level of success she hopes to is extremely important.

This highlights one of the many flaws we men possess, the inherent fact that if it's not important to us, then it must not be important to you. It is this misguided thinking that proves to get so many of us men in trouble and ultimately taking up residence in the metaphorical doghouse we are all too familiar with. Try to cut your knight in shining armor a little bit of slack though, ladies, for we know not what we do. It hasn't been without extreme patience and dedication that I have developed the internal dialogue I use on a daily basis to constantly remind myself that the relationship I'm in is not solely about me and the needs I require to be filled. There is in fact another human being needed to complete the equation of the relationship I desire to have. In this internal dialogue, I remind myself that she and the needs she possesses are just as equally important. I emphasize the truth that if I don't recognize this fact, I risk the vitality of the relationship I am in and may be destined for a lonely future. If I am not careful, the unfolding of my life will surely be filled with table settings for one at my favorite restaurants. I will be condemned to leave only a single set of footprints in the sands of the world's most exquisite beaches. I will ultimately be left alone with no partner, no companion to help construct the final memories used to write the closing chapters of my life.

It is my responsibility to recognize the gift she has actually given me. Here stands in front of me another human being committing herself to me. Unfortunately nowadays, with people changing in and out of relationships at the same rate they change the sheets on their bed, the concept of devoting your life to one other person holds none of the meaning it once did and should. When you actually stop to think about how truly special this concept is, it's mind-blowing to think of how lucky you should think of yourself in the event you find someone who is willing to do this, to devote his or her life to you! After all, each of us is given only one life, and the length of time our clock will tick is unknown. To think a woman would devote such a priceless and precious commodity to me is something that is so special, the words I strategically place together in an attempt to describe it will never be enough to properly define how extraordinary her gift truly is. Her offering should be treasured with more value placed on it than anything else I might stumble upon in life. Giving the gift of her precious and limited time on this earth and committing her efforts and energy to me is both profound and remarkable, and therefore should be continually treasured for what it is.

If I do set aside my ego and self-entitlement and put her needs in front of my own, I will always come out on top. It is through the desire and dedication of supporting my partner in reaching her goals that I can expect a truly profound change, or perhaps I should say lack of change in her. I get to wake up next to, live out my days with, and go to bed with the finest version of her. If I just lost any of you, what I mean to say is that each of us has different versions of ourselves. Versions that are happy, sad, frustrated or excited. We each also hold inside what I call the greatest version of ourselves — the one who is thirsty for life, happy-go-lucky, and extremely optimistic about every aspect of life. This is the same version that you present in the beginning stages of any relationship you've been in and the one that we men definitely fell for. I find the validity in my last statement to be ironic when I think about it. We men often complain, stating that our significant other has changed, that she's not the same person we met and fell in love with. The irony falls on the fact that this new person standing in front of us is a byproduct of our own faults, of our own continual and constant craving to always be right rather then seek an actual solution. In this case, the solution would be to set our own needs aside and support the needs of our partner.

In regard to her need to seek the physical transformation we have discussed throughout this book, I need to keep in the forefront of my mind that I am being given a tremendous opportunity. By supporting her on her journey rather than creating roadblocks for her to overcome, I essentially become a major source of positivity for her. I become the major building blocks she will need when constructing the ladder she will climb to reach her goals. Talk about putting myself in the best position possible. We all want to feel needed as human beings, right? Through my constant support, through my continual efforts to pick her up when she's fallen down, emerges a woman she never thought she could be.

As a backup plan in the event your Romeo doesn't share some of my unique perspectives in regard to relationships I will give you a Plan B.

Most of my clients have seen success in conversations related to support by validating the following facts: By improving her health and fitness level, she will be less stressed and better able to cope with challenging situations. In some cases, if she feels so inclined, I have had a few of the ladies throw a little icing on the cake by educating her special someone about a little physiological fact: the reality that consistent exercise has been shown to increases a female's sex drive! This is usually a sure way to seal the deal. Again, you know your partner better than anyone else, but I will tell you without question, the clients who have a willing counterpart in their journey reach profound levels of success compared with those who feel like they are all alone or, even worse, more of a burden during the process of reaching for their new goals.

For those of you who have children, this should be the point, age depending, you sit down with them and discuss what this new chapter of your life is all about, exactly how much it means to you, and how you need their help if you're going to make this happen. I've lost count of how many conversations I have had with mothers who were fear-stricken by the idea of their children finding out about their new lifestyle. Through the conversations I have had, it's fairly easy to tell they are fearful the child will feel neglected and less important, especially in the event the mom works full time and gets a limited amount of time with her children. It's easy to see how you can end up feeling bad about the idea of devoting any free time to activities outside work or your kids. I implore you to use the rest of this chapter and read what each of my clients' experiences have been to help ease your mind as well as enlighten you on exactly what effects your children will experience.

Let the record show that in all my clients' experiences, not a single child felt abandoned or unimportant after it was all said and done — not even one! In every case, the children were excited to hear the news. Most of the time they were thrilled by the idea of helping Mommy with something that is very special to her. It gives them a sense of importance and makes them feel needed, which is something we all want on a daily basis. Aside from these facts, there is a greater opportunity that presents itself in every single case. It's the opportunity to educate your children on valuable life lessons like self-respect and dedication. It's a chance to show them what it means to achieve what you're truly capable of despite what society says. It's the opportunity to show them just how strong their mother truly is and how much she is worth.

There is an interesting development that takes place, which

often comes as a big surprise to many of my clients. They are always shocked to see how invested their children become in their results. They find that by including the kids, they start to become their own personal little fan club! They tell Mommy positive things like how great she did in her workout today or how pretty she looks in her new clothes she was finally able to buy for herself. That said, they become your accountability team as well. They become direct with their questions like, "Aren't you suppose to be working out today?" in the event you decided to take a day off, or the famous question I hear they ask all the time, "Are you sure you're supposed to be eating that?" I personally love this because as a byproduct of taking control of your life and your potential, your children are becoming more aware. Aware of exactly how you got where you were and the negative impact it had on you, in turn, educating them on exactly what mistakes not to make themselves.

Let me share a personal story to help illustrate exactly how valuable these lessons will be for your children as they grow up. My childhood was not what most expected it would have been after meeting me. As I illustrated earlier in the book, I grew up with a mother who was a drug addict and alcoholic the majority of her life, and pretty much all of mine. My two younger siblings and I were witness to things that most adults never see, let alone young children. I have memories of waking up in the morning wondering why my mother hadn't come to wake us up, as she often did. I can recall the pit in my stomach after realizing this and searching the covers of our bed in a panic to make sure my sister and brother were both still safe with me. The three of us shared a bed at that time because we didn't have much money.

After ensuring they were safe, I quietly slipped out of bed so as not to wake them and began to search for my mother.

After scanning the upstairs of our apartment with no luck, I started walking down the stairs to search the main floor. That's when I found my mother face down on floor just in front of the stairs, lying in her own vomit. She had clearly partied a little to hard, to put it mildly, and after passing out must have aspirated while facedown. At no more than the age of six or seven, I was forced to roll her over onto her back because I wasn't sure if she was still breathing or if she had choked to death. I have memories of watching my mother doze off at the dinner table from whatever prescription-medication cocktail she had taken prior to us all sitting down as a family to eat. I could see the looks of confusion and concern from my sister and brother, so I did the most logical thing at the time and lied to them when they asked, "Why doesn't Mom stay awake to eat with us?" or "Should we take Mom's food away so she doesn't choke?" Often my response was simply that she was just sleepy because she needed a new mattress and therefore wasn't sleeping well.

The list of my experiences like these goes on to the point that I could quite possibly double the size of this book, but that's not its point. Those of you thinking how awful this must have been for a young child to experience, I would agree, in the moment, yes, it was a difficult time for me. Especially at an age when I was not yet able to rationalize with why my mother's choices didn't include her being the mother to us I desperately wanted her to. The kind of mother so many of my friends had. The point of this little glimpse into my history is not for you to feel sorry for me. I told you these stories to point out that it was these very experiences that molded me into who I am today with the lessons they provided. For friends of mine who do know my past, I often tell them these experiences were in fact one of the greatest gifts my mother had ever given to me, because despite all that I didn't understand, the one thing I knew beyond a doubt was that I never wanted to subject myself or my own family to that lifestyle or those experiences.

As I grew up, this made the time when so many of my peers were choosing to experiment with drugs and alcohol an easy choice for me. While so many of them were making poor choices out of either pure pressure or just simple curiosity, I found that equipped with the memories I had filed away from my childhood, I had no interest in drugs and alcohol. I didn't possess the normal curiosity that kids have at that age that keeps so many parents up at night, and it was because of my past. Despite the fact that most of you would consider the comparison of drug and alcohol abuse to a few extra pounds around the midsection completely absurd, I feel that depends on who you talk to and what their definition of addiction is.

After all, a few extra pounds in almost all cases is related to an inability to step away from the fridge when you should; it is an addiction. The only difference between being addicted to drugs and alcohol or foods you shouldn't be consuming on a regular basis is, quite frankly, the speed at which they kill you. With studies showing an unquestionable connection between the foods we eat and the way we eat them, and the metabolically driven diseases that are killing us daily, you would be hard-pressed to rationalize the fact that living in an obese state is the less harmful option. Perhaps the comparison isn't so far off when you look at it through a different lens.

Back to the immeasurable opportunity you have as a mother to educate those kids and potentially alter their path or standard they keep for their own personal health. That brings up very valid point I want to make. For a moment I want you to think in the context of your own childhood and the habits you have today that have put you where you're at physically when you look in the mirror. Looking at those habits, I would bet money on the fact that most of them were not self-taught. I would venture to guess you didn't develop a love of Doritos as a toddler by opening the pantry door, climbing up to the third shelf and ripping open a fresh bag thinking, "Hmmm... I think I'll try some Doritos today!" Absolutely not. Instead, you were fed them on a consistent-enough basis to develop a taste for them by your parents. This is not to say they were planning to make your life more difficult with a fierce love of Doritos; it was more or less just a lack of education on their part. Think of all it could have prevented in your life if they had the knowledge you now possess! I discuss this topic with virtually every one of the women I work with.

Now that we have covered some key facts to touch on when asking your other half for a little extra support and hopefully given you a different viewpoint in relation to the effects your journey will have on your children, let's get into the reason why not dealing with your emotional triggers is a far bigger issue than you think.

If you're trying to answer that question yourself after reading this chapter, the answer should be outlined pretty easily. Not dealing with your emotional triggers will cause you to fail! Yes, this is true, but you're missing half of the statement. It should read: "Not dealing with your emotional triggers will cause you to fail *before you even get started!*" And that is the bigger issue. In case you don't recall, I already outlined how failure is not final, and therefore, not a big deal. Nor is it the end of the world. You can work to overcome failure; you can pick up the pieces and keep moving forward. Where I see the major difference between my clients who succeed and those who absolutely crash and burn is at which stage they fail. I will say it again because it's so important to fully grasp: The stage in which you fail will dictate your outcome.

Let's take a moment to illustrate this. If you ever meet a trainer or another woman in the gym who states that every day of their fitness journey has been the greatest experience of their lives, you need to immediately squirt them directly in the face with your water bottle, call them a liar, and walk away. For me and all of my clients, not one of us have had nothing but rainbows and unicorns every single day since we started our journeys to hitting our fitness goals. It simply doesn't happen. That's not to say that some days aren't truly great, because they are, and you should expect plenty of them, but you will have off-days. Days when you look in the mirror and try to recall the watermelon you clearly swallowed the day before. You're going to have days when an emotional trigger is getting the best of you. The most useful tool you have in that situation is time, aka skin in the game. If you're not where you want to be yet physically, but you have dropped sixty or seventy pounds of fat off your body, the odds are when you get up to look in the mirror, you're going to be reminded of how much time or skin in the game you have. That in my experience has been enough

The Woman Missing In The Mirror

to push my clients to that workout they were considering skipping.

Now let's look at the other side of the coin. Let's say you're a week into your program, so you have not yet seen any physical changes (which you shouldn't) and — boom! — you're hit with an emotional trigger. Your husband or special someone kept you up all night snoring or one of the kids is sick. Odds are when you look in the mirror and see no change, you'll end up filling your head with reasons why it's pointless to force yourself to go to the gym, such as you're not making changes anyway so you decide to skip that day. In most cases, I watch that one day turn into two days, then one week, and eventually you come to terms with the fact that you're going to be out of shape forever. Again, the only thing different by comparison between the two clients is one has stuck it out long enough to witness physical changes (has some skin in the game), while other has not. It has nothing to do with one being more physically capable than the other. What I want you to take away from this is, it actually gets easier to stay on track the longer you do it. But the beginning is by far the most challenging, and therefore a crucial time of your journey.

163

TESTIMONIAL

Five years ago after having back surgery I gained 30 pounds and was left with neuropathy from my knee down on the right side of my right leg. I was very stiff in all my joints, my knees are now bone on bone and in need of knee replacement . I was unable to squat or do a lunge. After working with Dean I have lost 20 pounds and my joints feel much for flexible. This was the first time in my life that I have lost weight and not gained. The diet was easy to follow. Dean will tell you when to eat, what to eat, and how much you can eat and I never felt hungry. Last week for the first time I was able to do a squat and a lunge without holding onto anything!!

Sincerely Lory

What we think, we become.

—*Buddha*

10:
PROJECTING TO
THE FINISH LINE

Take it from me: This next topic is in relation to something even the best of us experience, including myself. I believe it to be in our nature as human beings to be discontent. We often criticize ourselves and the fact that we have yet to accomplish all we had hoped for. Regardless of whether we are discussing finances, your current occupation or, in the case of this book, your current physical state, it matters nonetheless. In one or all of these examples, it would be easy to tally a monstrous list of individuals who are unhappy or despondent when asked how they feel about those aspects of their lives. Perhaps he or she had expectations of capturing a few more zeros for their bank account by now. Or maybe they anticipated having moved out of that tiny cubicle by now that leaves them feeling claustrophobic and into that spacious office that includes an actual window and a fancy nameplate on the door with their first and last name accompanied by the extraordinary words "Executive Account Manager."

Or perchance you're simply like so many of the women I have helped throughout the years. You spend your days with a paralyzing feeling of desolation every time you stand in front of that mirror! You know with every thread of your being that the woman staring back shares no resemblance to the woman who is trapped beneath it all. As if the beautiful, sexy and vibrant woman you truly are has been locked away deep inside the complete stranger you now present to the world. In any of these cases, there is always a strong yearning for change that develops when having these feelings of displeasure, unhappiness or the overwhelming feeling of being inadequate. For purposes of the scope of this book, we will continue our discussion under the assumption you're one of the many woman who are desperate for physical changes.

As your yearning for this change is inevitably fed by all of the powerful negative emotions we just touched on, there is an additional underlying issue that is created. As your craving for change grows, so does the desire to see these changes happen overnight. This desire for overnight success has proved to be the root of all evil, and when rooted too deeply, has the power to destroy even my most committed clients. It is for this reason that I discuss timelines with each and every woman I sit down with. In my initial discussions with a potential client, I always ask her what kind of timeline she has in mind to reach her goals. Inevitably, the timeline she gives is much too short. This needs to be addressed immediately because it can create a false set of expectations she never should have had in the first place. This brings me to one of the main points of this chapter: Do not prepare yourself to run a one-hundred-yard dash when you're actually about to run a long-distance marathon. Obviously the distance you will ultimately need to run in this metaphorical race depends greatly on how considerable the physical changes are you require.

So how do so many of you end up running the wrong race?

It's a byproduct of the fitness industry and consumers being desperate for instant gratification or overnight success. Essentially the masterminds behind the massive companies responsible for the development of the countless products and workout options you now have got hip to the fact that if they invent something that fulfills your desire for instant success, then their wallets are going to be a whole lot fatter at the end of the year. Aside from filling some pockets with your hard-earned money, you can also expect to develop a tremendously strong expectation for extremely quick results.

Let's use the extremely popular example of twenty- and thirty-day challenges that I read so much about and see so many of you gravitating toward. They make claims that in twenty or thirty days, you can expect to lose ten, twenty or even thirty pounds in this short amount of time. With claims like this, you would have to be crazy not to jump on the bandwagon! Unfortunately, most of you haven't been trained to properly read between the lines. Stop for a second and ask yourself what these different companies, fitness centers and even personal trainers are claiming the results are you can expect. They claim that in twenty or thirty days, you can lose ten, twenty or even thirty pounds. Did you catch the magic word they are using? That you will lose ten, twenty or even thirty *pounds*.

With the education and principles I have now equipped you with, the question you should immediately ask is, "If I chose to participate in this challenge, I should plan to lose ten, twenty or even thirty pounds of what?" You'd better hope you're not losing ten, twenty or thirty pounds of that precious muscle you now know is the stuff that doesn't jiggle or fall to the floor when your clothes do. It's the stuff that leaves you feeling confident when you step out into the sunshine and onto that sandy beach in your favorite two-piece bathing suit. It's that golden ticket, that magic metabolism you finally hold in your possession that allows you to sleep like a baby after a night filled with delicious foods and strong drinks knowing you will undoubtedly wake to find those slender lines and sexy curves smiling back at you in the mirror the next morning. You better hope you're not losing the ten, twenty or thirty pounds of muscle that is, in fact ,the holy grail of your long-term success. Remembering the statement I made earlier in this book that muscle is three times denser than fat, this essentially means it is three times heavier from a scale standpoint. In knowing this information, you'll realize that products, workouts and diets are developed with the sole purpose of going after as much of your beloved muscle as possible. After all, up to the point you purchased this book, you too were probably fixated on the scale and the number it spit back at you, just like nine out of ten other women walking around the streets are today. With this formula in mind, it makes complete sense why products like the ones I have described come to exist. If that product can produce a significant reduction in your muscle, that muscle that is three times heavier on the scale, the outcome will not only be a drastic decrease in scale weight, but a rapid one at that.

This leaves anyone who decided to utilize these particular products, workouts or diets with a false sense of success. Despite the fact that the number on the scale has dropped notably, the only true results they have been left with is a metabolism that can support minimal calories at best and zero room for error in the kitchen. In this position, one night out on the town for this poor woman would surely prove to be catastrophic. This squandering of her precious muscle will also prove to leave her with a physical appearance reflecting nothing she had hoped for. She will inevitably be left with soft, squishy and sagging body parts.

This helps to illustrate how and why so many of you end up in that dark abyss filled with hopelessness, defeat, discouragement and despair. You live a life of performing the same delicate dance day in and day out. Avoiding all your favorite foods at all costs as if they were the Black Plague, assuming food is what's making you fat, when actually it's your missing metabolism that's behind it all. Miserably forcing yourself into gyms or programs that offer highly intense and highly dangerous workouts designed for elite athletes in hopes of burning colossal amounts of calories and, in turn, finally ridding yourself of that unsightly body fat, a setting you now know to be far too intense to target body fat. I have also illustrated why so many of you live in fear of changing any of your current practices or habits. You feel as if you're hanging on by a mere thread to a body you really don't approve of as it is, but don't dare risk the potential of taking any more steps in the wrong direction.

Herein lies the issue. These products that I described as being developed with the intention of putting you in the fragile state we just discussed are also developed with the interest of keeping you dependent on them. Talk about a brilliant business model! They sell you something that makes you look and feel good only for the amount of time you use it. Think in terms of illness and the different medications you can take for them. Would you choose the medicine that masks your symptoms but offers no actual cure, forcing you to live out your days dependent on it? Or would you opt for the remedy that, when taken properly for the right amount of time, will rid your body of that illness forever? I won't claim to know the option you would chose, but I will tell you this book was written to offer you the same antidote that each of the ladies I have worked with has been given. The same antidote that has proved to cure them of an illness they were certain they would suffer from for the rest of their lives. For a moment, though, imagine if things were different for you. Imagine if by just sticking to the set of key principles I have provided you with in this book you will never again have to rely on a bottle of weight-loss pills, some screwball workout, or crash diet. Imagine how marvelous you will feel knowing all you need to depend on is yourself to transform any part of your body. Talk about feeling empowered. Talk about a future of limitless physical potential!

Now that we have addressed how so many of you have developed false ideas of how long it should actually take you to achieve your own personal transformation, let's discuss how to set the right timeline for your goal.

Regardless of who my client is or what her personal goals are, I start all of them out on a twelve-week timeline. The reason for this length of time I choose to start at is for two main reasons. Remember my expectations for each of you, as it has been with everyone of my clients, is for you to not only achieve the level of success you had hoped for, but to along the way have also created a new set of habits. The set of habits that will carry you through life and all of its twists and turns with the ability to maintain your success for the rest of your life. As I often say: Getting women results is the easy part; giving them the skills to maintain them for a lifetime is the greater triumph. I find that within the first twelve weeks, we have restructured and replaced habits as well as worked our way through any initial stages that might require a bit of a learning curve. Some of the emotional attachments you have to the habits we are attempting to reformat or possibly even replace completely might prove to be stronger than expected and therefore require a few gentle nudges along the way. Once habitual behaviors have been reprogrammed, this is the point I see my clients really begin to take flight and soar away from those dark, somber, rain-filled skies and into the warm sunlight of success.

At this point, timelines pivot solely on the amount of physical change you wish to attain. If you're like some of my clients who came to me with hopes of dropping a mere dress size or simply tightening things up, I would venture to say these type of results should be expected in three to six months. In the event you're like many of my other personal clients who hired me to accomplish what was assumed impossible, one who seeks a transformation so dramatic that it's highly probably most people wouldn't recognize you in the event you actually attained this paramount goal. I will ask you to keep something in mind. Undoubtedly the inches you wish to lose didn't find their way onto you in a matter of weeks, or even months. For reasons that should hold little relevance to you at this point, the inches or body fat I am referring to have been allowed to collect and compile most likely for years. Having expectations of eliminating them in a few measly months is not only unrealistic but, more important, it's a sure-fire way to set yourself up for monumental disappointment when you fail to hit a goal you never stood a chance of hitting in the first place. This section of the chapter was by no means intended to discourage you.

I feel that regardless of how sore this subject is, the sooner we establish the race you're actually running, the sooner we can put you on the fast track to finally crossing that finish line.

Here is the light at the end of the tunnel that I hope you use to help rekindle your flames of fortitude. In more than fifteen years of training a multitude of female clients, all seeking unique results, including the most basic physical changes to the most climactic physical transformations one can conceive, I have yet to meet a single woman I could not guide to the finish line when she followed the principles I have outlined in this book. The only times I have seen women waiver from the success they're capable of is when they create false expectations of when they feel they should cross that finish line. Using the illustration of illness and medication again, imagine you've gone to your primary-care doctor because you are suffering from an illness. After an initial exam and diagnosis, your doctor informs you that you need to take a specific medication for a total of six weeks, and you should find yourself at that point finally starting to feel better. Despite the fact you were keeping your fingers crossed for a quicker recovery, you take the advice of your doctor and follow through with his recommendations, eventually recovering. Why in this circumstance did you not decide your doctor is in fact mental and tell yourself you will be fully recovered in two weeks, tops? Despite your desire to heal much quicker, you simply accept the reality of your situation. Why should your ability to make the physical transformation you seek be any different? Despite your desperate desire to finally see the woman in the mirror who's been hidden for so long, you owe it to yourself to be rational rather than emotional.

A key component to your continued success now and through the years to come is having the expectation in the back of your mind that those dark, gloomy, rain-filled skies you know all to well might reappear from time to time. Be prepared to weather the storm. As is always the case, the storm will pass, and those blue skies and warm rays of sunshine will be close behind. I find it's my less-seasoned clients who forget this little tip and fall apart at the first sign of trouble. Remember, if the physical changes you seek were attained easily or required only a small amount of effort, everyone would look amazing, I would be unemployed, and there would be no need for a book like this to be written. Be tenacious in your efforts to stay on track during the more-challenging days, and you will come out smelling like a rose every time.

TESTIMONIAL

About two and half years ago I quit my job as an executive at a major automotive company after 32 years in the business. I was exhausted, out of shape, and unhappy with myself. I realized it was time to take charge of my life and make a change. This was a huge step, because I walked away from everything I'd known — my job was my identity and it was all consuming. It had become so demanding that after years of being committed to daily exercise, I found myself lucky to get in 2-3 days on the elliptical in a week. I was sleep deprived and not happy. So I took the leap, stopped working, and started creating a new life including fitness. However, I found that exercise wasn't enough to get me where I wanted to be. It was shortly after realizing this that I hired Dean and began his Program. After changing both my fitness regimen and my eating habits, I started to notice changes happening in the direction I wanted. I also noticed I was sleeping better, and felt better both mentally and physically. I had more energy, and my family began commenting on how I smiled and laughed more and seem genuinely happy. About a year ago I went back to work part time in a less demanding role, which provides some mental stimulation and supports my fitness habit. Dean's principles have successfully taught me how to manage my nutrition and fitness effectively and have really made a difference in my outlook on life!

Susan

It is never too late to be what you might have been.

—*George Eliot*

11:
FINAL THOUGHTS TO CARRY WITH YOU

I will close this book with a message that I hope resonates with you for the days, weeks, months and years to come. My aspirations are that through this book you have finally come to realize your true beauty. I sincerely hope you remind yourself each and every day who is actually reflecting back when you look in the mirror. No matter how long the woman has been missing in the mirror, regardless of the length of time she has been hidden from the world, she still stands right in front of you reflecting back. The woman who's merely a distant memory at this point, buried beneath countless years of tried-and-failed attempts, encased in a tomb of hopelessness, depression and despair, still remains. Hiding underneath the enormous scar you bare as a reminder of countless moments and experiences filled with embarrassment, difficulty and discouragement still resides that perfect version of you. I sincerely hope you constantly remind yourself of the undeniable fact that you are the beautiful and priceless painting described in the beginning of this book. Always remembering your value is truly immeasurable. Regardless of your age or body type, you are priceless and absolutely worth it!

You're not just that single mom or housewife whose identity can be found only in her function of making sure her husband and children are well cared for, the dishes are done, your dinners are cooked, and the house is neatly kept. You're not just that businesswoman whose only objective in life is to become a valued asset to the company and climb to the highest levels of the proverbial corporate ladder before you hopefully make it to retirement without dying first. My hope is that each of you has cultivated the same lens I look through every time I meet a woman for the first time. It is through this lens that I see her true elegance, her true beauty and her limitless potential. I see the woman she thought had vanished long ago smiling back at me! Every second, every moment and every day is an opportunity to apply the principles I have provided for you. Take back your life, the life that somehow slipped through your fingers when you weren't looking. Despite what you see in the mirror, that woman you're searching for is there underneath it all. Underneath the doubt, underneath the fear, underneath the hopelessness, she's right in front of you, waiting to finally reflect back when you step in front of that mirror!

ABOUT THE AUTHOR

Dean Mitchell is an entrepreneur, author, and health and wellness expert who has found extreme success through working exclusively with women all over the country to help them achieve the unachievable. With his career in the fitness industry dating back to the better part of fifteen years, it's easy to understand how he's held every position imaginable. From scrubbing floors and fitness equipment to managing the day-to-day operations of big-box clubs, he eventually settled into his current position as a consultant for women throughout the country. He is the co-founder of Mitchell Fitness Solutions, his premier training facility that is one-hundred percent personalized to fit his clients individual needs.

Despite the success Dean has achieved in his career, his personal life includes a dark past that most are shocked to learn about. Starting out life without his biological father and with a mother who struggled with mental illness and drug addiction, he and his two siblings grew up in a poverty-stricken environment filled with chaos and turmoil. With his mother struggling to care for herself, let alone her children, he recalls being forced to grow up extremely quickly to tend to his mother's and younger siblings' needs. Despite his challenging beginnings, life has continued to test his will through experiences with tragedy and loss that most of us only read about. A few of Dean's "tests," as he calls them, include his mother suffering a massive stroke that would leave her partially paralyzed without the use of one side of her body at the young age of forty-four. The loss of both his siblings through suicide and a drug overdose are just a few more examples of what he has had to overcome before reaching his mid-thirties.

Despite being faced with adversity that would force most to throw in the towel, it is Dean's insatiable desire to help others that has kept him focused on his life's purpose. His latest project is his first book, *The Woman Missing in the Mirror,* which is about to go into presale. He hopes through his book's release it will help extend his reach even farther, making him an ambassador for women throughout the world, convincing them of the true potential they posses by giving them the same set of his unique principles he's provided each of his clients that has allowed so many to see their true potential and how limitless it is.

To receive one of Dean's personalized nutrition programs for FREE just follow these two steps!

First, go to www.DeanPMitchell.com and register to join his rapidly growing community of women who have found the woman missing in the mirror.

Next, simply share a selfie of you with your copy of *The Woman Missing In The Mirror* on your Facebook and or Instagram pages or share this video (vimeo. com/181718968) on your Facebook page. Be sure to tag the author and include the hashtag *#ifoundher* !

CONNECT WITH THE AUTHOR

Location:
Dean Mitchell Owner/CEO
Mitchell Fitness Solutions
133 W. Main St STE 240
Northville, MI 48167

Website:
www.DeanPMitchell.com

Email:
deanomitchell16@gmail.com

Social Media:
www.facebook.com/DeanPMitchell
www.instagram.com/deanpmitchell
www.twitter.com/mitchell2426